Lecture Notes on Haematology

Lecture Notes on Haematology

N.C. HUGHES-JONES

DM, PhD, MA, FRCP, FRS
Honorary Member of the Scientific Staff,
Medical Research Council's
Molecular Immunopathology Unit;
Visiting Professor,
Department of Haematology,
St Mary's Hospital Medical School,
Norfolk Place, London;
Member of the
Department of Pathology,
University of Cambridge

S.N. WICKRAMASINGHE

ScD, PhD, MB BS, FRCPath, MRCP, FIBiol
Professor of Haematology
in the University of London;
Head of the Department of Haematology,
St Mary's Hospital Medical School,
Imperial College of Science, Technology and Medicine,
Norfolk Place, London;
Honorary Consultant Haematologist,
Parkside Health Authority, London

FIFTH EDITION

OXFORD

BLACKWELL SCIENTIFIC PUBLICATIONS

LONDON EDINBURGH BOSTON

MELBOURNE PARIS BERLIN VIENNA

© 1970, 1973, 1979, 1984, 1991 by
Blackwell Scientific Publications
Editorial Offices:
Osney Mead, Oxford OX2 0EL
25 John Street, London WC1N 2BL
23 Ainslie Place, Edinburgh EH3 6AJ
3 Cambridge Center, Cambridge
  Massachusetts 02142, USA
54 University Street, Carlton
  Victoria 3053, Australia

Other Editorial Offices:
Arnette SA
2, rue Casimir-Delavigne
75006 Paris
France

Blackwell Wissenschaft
Meinekestrasse 4
D–1000 Berlin 15
Germany

Blackwell MZV
Feldgasse 13
A–1238 Wien
Austria

First published 1970
Second edition 1973
Reprinted 1975
Third edition 1979
Reprinted 1980
Fourth edition 1984
Fifth edition 1991

Set by Times Graphics, Singapore
Printed and bound in Great Britain
at the Alden Press, Oxford

DISTRIBUTORS
Marston Book Services Ltd
PO Box 87
Oxford OX2 0DT
(*Orders*: Tel. 0865 791155
         Fax: 0865 791927
         Telex: 837515)

USA
Mosby-Year Book, Inc.
11830 Westline Industrial Drive
St Louis, Missouri 63146
(*Orders*: Tel: 800 633–6699)

Canada
Mosby-Year Book, Inc.
5240 Finch Avenue East
Scarborough, Ontario
(*Orders*: Tel: (416) 298–1588)

Australia
Blackwell Scientific Publications
(Australia) Pty Ltd
54 University Street
Carlton, Victoria 3053
(*Orders*: Tel: (03) 347–0300)

British Library
Cataloguing in Publication Data

Hughes-Jones, N. C. (Nevin Campbell)
1923–
   Lecture notes on haematology
   5th ed.
   1. Medicine. Haematology
   I. Title   II. Wickramasinghe, S. N.
(Sunitha Nimal)   616.15

ISBN 0-632-02768-1

Contents

Preface to Fifth Edition

In this edition we have re-written and updated many sections of the book. In addition we have included a chapter on myeloma and lymphomas. The basic purpose of this volume remains the same as that of the first edition, namely to provide core knowledge in haematology both for the medical student and the newly-qualified doctor. Unfortunately, as in many other subjects in medicine, there is no uniformly accepted view of what constitutes core knowledge, and some departments teach certain topics in much greater detail than others. In order that the book will be useful to most students, we have included some information that we do not ourselves consider to be core knowledge but which we know is taught in some schools; such information is presented but not discussed in any detail.

A new feature of this edition is the inclusion of 32 colour plates illustrating various aspects of normal and abnormal blood and bone marrow smears. We are grateful to Immuno AG, Immuno Limited, Celltech and Sandoz Pharmaceuticals for so generously sponsoring the colour plates. We also thank Drs A. Zuiable and S. H. Abdalla for providing material for some of the plates and the Audio-Visual Department of St Mary's Hospital Medical School for permission to reproduce the clinical illustrations.

N. C. Huges-Jones
S. N. Wickramasinghe

Preface to First Edition

These lecture notes are designed to supply the basic knowledge of both the clinical and laboratory aspects of haematological diseases and blood transfusion. The content is broadly similar to that of the course given to medical students by the Department of Haematology at St Mary's Hospital Medical School. References have been cited so that those who need to extend their knowledge in any particular field can do so. Most of the journals and books that are mentioned are those commonly found in every library.

At the end of each chapter I have supplied a list of objectives in studying each disease. There are two main purposes in these objectives. First, they facilitate the learning process, since the process of acquisition, retention and recall of data is greatly helped if the facts and concepts are centred around a particular objective. Secondly, many objectives are closely related to the practical problems encountered in the diagnosis and treatment of patients. For instance, the following objectives: 'to understand the method of differentiation of megaloblastic anaemia due to Vitamin B_{12} deficiency from that due to folate deficiency' and 'to understand the basis for the differentiation of leukaemia into acute and chronic forms based on the clinical picture and on the peripheral blood findings' are practical problems encountered frequently in the haematology laboratory. A point of more immediate interest to the undergraduate is that examiners setting either multiple choice or essay questions will be searching for the same knowledge that is required in answering the objectives.

I should like to thank Professor P. L. Mollison, Dr P. Barkhan, Dr I. Chanarin, Dr G. J. Jenkins and Dr M. S. Rose for their criticism and helpful suggestions during the preparation of the manuscript and Mrs Inge Barnett for typing the several drafts and final typescript.

N. C. Hughes-Jones

Chapter 1
Haemopoiesis and Blood Cells

INTRAUTERINE HAEMOPOIESIS AND POSTNATAL CHANGES

The production of blood cells (haemopoiesis) begins in the yolk sac of the 14–19 day human embryo. The fetal liver becomes the main site of haemopoiesis in the second trimester of pregnancy and the fetal bone marrow in the third trimester. The majority of the haemopoietic cells in the yolk sac and fetal liver are erythroblasts. The main site of granulocytopoietic activity in intrauterine life is the fetal bone marrow. Some characteristics of intrauterine erythropoiesis are summarized in Table 1.1.

After birth, the marrow is the sole site of haemopoiesis in healthy individuals. During the first 4 years of life, nearly all the marrow cavities contain red haemopoietic marrow with very few fat cells. Thereafter, increasing numbers of fat cells appear in certain marrow cavities. By the age of 25 years, the only sites of active haemopoiesis are the skull bones, ribs, sternum, scapulae, clavicles, vertebrae, pelvis, the upper half of the sacrum and the proximal ends of the shafts of the femur and humerus. All the remaining marrow cavities contain yellow fatty marrow. Even at sites of active haemopoiesis, about half the volume of the marrow normally consists of fat cells.

In a number of diseases (e.g. chronic haemolytic anaemias, megaloblastic anaemias and some leukaemias) there may be (a) a partial or complete replacement of fat cells by haemopoietic cells in marrow cavities normally supporting haemopoiesis; (b) extension of haemopoietic marrow into marrow cavities normally containing non-haemopoietic fatty marrow (e.g. in long bones); and (c) the appearance of foci of haemopoietic tissue in the liver and spleen (extramedullary haemopoiesis).

Table 1.1 Some characteristics of intrauterine erythropoiesis.

Site of erythropoiesis	Predominant type of erythropoiesis	End-cell	Main types of haemoglobin
Yolk sac	Megaloblastic	Nucleated	Gower 1, $(\zeta_2\varepsilon_2)$ Gower II, $(\alpha_2\varepsilon_2)$ Portland I, $(\zeta_2\gamma_2)$
Fetal liver	Normoblastic	Anucleate, macrocytes	Fetal haemoglobin (HbF, $\alpha_2\gamma_2$)
Fetal bone marrow	Normoblastic	Anucleate, macrocytes	HbF, and HbA $(\alpha_2\beta_2)$

HAEMOPOIESIS IN THE ADULT

General considerations and early events

Haemopoietic systems of adults are examples of steady-state cell renewal systems in which the rate of loss of mature cells (red cells, granulocytes, monocytes, lymphocytes and platelets) from the blood is balanced fairly precisely by the rate of release of newly formed cells into the blood. Mature cells are lost either because of ageing or during the performance of normal functions.

The formation of blood cells involves two processes:

1   progressive development of structural and functional characteristics specific for a given cell type (cytodifferentiation or maturation);

2   cell proliferation.

A schematic representation of haemopoiesis is shown in Fig. 1.1. The stem cells and progenitor cells involved in haemopoiesis cannot be recognized morphologically in marrow smears but can be studied by functional tests. In man, these cells (colony-forming units or CFU) have been identified and characterized on the basis of their ability to produce small colonies of one or more cell types when grown in semi-solid media containing appropriate haemopoietic growth factors. The most primitive haemopoietic cell is the pluripotent haemopoietic stem cell. This gives rise to two types of committed stem cell, namely multipotent myeloid stem cells and lymphoid stem cells. Stem cells have an extensive capacity to maintain their own number by cell proliferation in addition to the capacity to mature into other cell types. The lymphoid stem cells give rise to lymphocyte progenitor cells that eventually mature into all types of T, B and non-T, non-B lymphocyte. The multipotent myeloid stem cells differentiate into various types of myeloid progenitor cell which eventually generate erythrocytes, neutrophils, eosinophils, basophils and mast cells, monocytes and platelets. Unlike the stem cells, the lymphoid and myeloid progenitor cells have only a limited capacity for self-renewal. The more immature myeloid progenitor cells are committed to two or three differentiation pathways. With increasing maturity, their differentiation potential becomes progressively limited, eventually to one pathway only. The unipotent progenitor cells committed to the production of erythrocytes, neutrophil granulocytes, monocytes/macrophages and megakaryocytes are, respectively, called CFU-E, CFU-G, CFU-M and CFU-mega. They mature into the earliest morphologically recognizable cells of the corresponding cell lineage (pronormoblasts, myeloblasts, monoblasts and megakaryoblasts).

Morphologically recognizable haemopoietic cells derived from myeloid stem cells

In every myeloid cell lineage other than that involved in platelet production, the early precursors that can be identified on morphological and cytochemical criteria are capable of both dividing and maturing. The late precursors do not divide but continue to mature. The proliferative activity during haemopoiesis serves as an amplifying mechanism and ensures that a large number of mature blood cells is derived from a single cell that becomes committed to any particular lineage. The lack of cell division in megakaryocytes is discussed later.

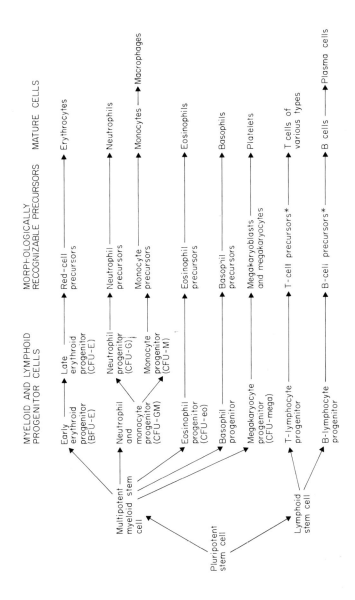

*Identification based not on morphology but on immunochemical and gene re-arrangement criteria

Fig. 1.1   Relationships between the various types of cell involved in haemopoiesis.

Erythropoiesis

The pronormoblast is a large cell with a small quantity of agranular intensely basophilic cytoplasm (due to the presence of numerous ribosomes) and a large nucleus containing finely-dispersed nuclear chromatin and nucleoli (Fig. 1.2a. The successive stages through which a pronormoblast develops into erythrocytes are termed basophilic normoblasts (Fig. 1.2b); early and late polychromatic normoblasts (Fig. 1.2c, d); and marrow reticulocytes and blood reticulocytes. Nucleated cell classes of increasing maturity show (a) a progressive reduction in cell and nuclear size; (b) a progressive increase in the quantity of condensed nuclear chromatin; (c) a progressive increase in the ratio of cytoplasmic volume to nuclear volume; and (d) a progressive increase in haemoglobin (which stains pink) and a progressive decrease in ribosomal RNA (which stains blue), resulting

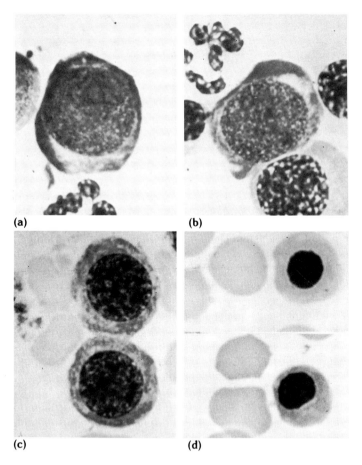

(a)   (b)

(c)   (d)

Fig. 1.2 (a) Pronormoblast. (b) Basophilic normoblast. (c) Two early polychromatic normoblasts. (d) Two late polychromatic normoblasts. The granules of condensed chromatin in the basophilic normoblast are slightly coarser than in the pronormoblast. The nuclei of the late polychromatic normoblasts contain large masses of condensed chromatin.

in polychromasia. The late polychromatic normoblast extrudes its nucleus and becomes a marrow reticulocyte. The marrow reticulocytes enter the blood stream and circulate for 1–2 days before becoming mature red cells.

In Romanowsky-stained marrow and blood smears, reticulocytes appear as rounded, faintly polychromatic, cells whose diameters are slightly larger than those of mature red cells. When living polychromatic red cells are incubated with brilliant cresyl blue (supravital staining), the ribosomes form a basophilic precipitate of granules or filaments; in the most immature of these cells the precipitated RNA appears as a basophilic reticulum (hence the term reticulocyte) (Fig. 1.3). Mature red cells lack ribosomes.

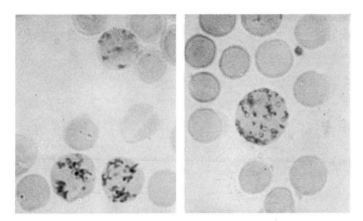

Fig. 1.3 Reticulocytes in peripheral blood stained supravitally with brilliant cresyl blue. Note the reticulum of precipitated ribosomes.

On the basis of their morphological features, nucleated red-cell precursors (erythroblasts) found in normal marrow are called normoblasts and normal erythropoiesis is described as being normoblastic in type. The characteristic feature of normoblastic erythropoiesis is the presence of moderate quantities of condensed nuclear chromatin in early polychromatic erythroblasts.

Even in healthy individuals, a few erythroblasts fail to develop normally and such cells are recognized and phagocytosed by bone marrow macrophages. This loss of potential erythrocytes due to the intramedullary destruction of red cell precursors is described as ineffective erythropoiesis. The extent of ineffective erythropoiesis in normal marrow is slight.

Neutrophil granulocytopoiesis

The myeloblasts superficially resemble pronormoblasts except that their cytoplasm is less basophilic. The successive cytological classes through which a myeloblast matures into circulating neutrophil granulocytes are termed promyelocytes, neutrophil myelocytes, neutrophil metamyelocytes and marrow neutrophil granulocytes (Fig. 1.4, Plates 1–3). During this maturation the following changes occur:

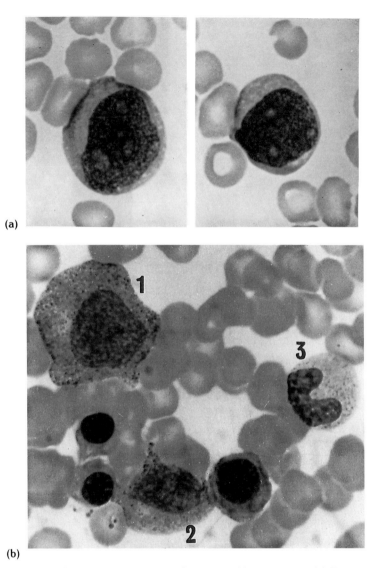

Fig. 1.4 Neutrophil precursors from normal bone marrow. (a) Two myeloblasts. (b) Promyelocyte (1) myelocyte (2) and metamyelocyte (3).

1 a progressive reduction of cytoplasmic basophilia and a progressive increase in the quantity of condensed chromatin after the promyelocyte stage;

2 the formation of coarse purplish-red (azurophilic) cytoplasmic granules (primary granules) at the promyelocyte stage, which remain visible at the myelocyte stage but not later;

3 the formation of fine neutrophilic granules (specific granules) at the myelocyte and metamyelocyte stages;

4 moderate indentation of the nucleus at the metamyelocyte stage (which is characterized by a C- or U-shaped nucleus);

5 progressive segmentation of the U-shaped nucleus at the granulocyte stage until it consists of 2–5 lobes.

Megakaryocytopoiesis

During megakaryocytopoiesis, there is replication of DNA without nuclear or cell division which leads to the generation of very large uninucleate cells with DNA contents between 8C and 64C (other haemopoietic cells have DNA contents between 2C and 4C). There is a rough correlation between the DNA content of a megakaryocyte nucleus and both its size and extent of lobulation. A mature megakaryocyte is illustrated in Fig. 1.5 and in Plate 4. Large numbers of

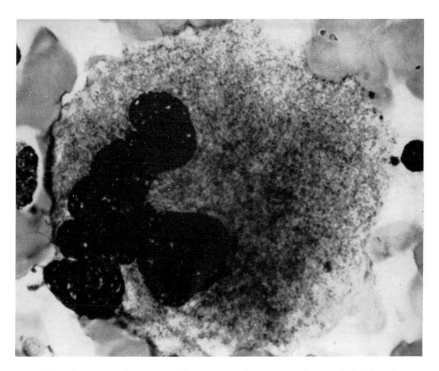

Fig. 1.5 Mature megakaryocyte. This is a very large cell with a single lobulated nucleus. Compare the size of the megakaryocyte with that of the neutrophil granulocyte and lymphocyte nearby.

platelets are formed from the cytoplasm of each mature megakaryocyte; these are rapidly discharged directly into the marrow sinusoids. The residual 'bare' megakaryocyte nucleus is phagocytosed by macrophages.

Monocytopoiesis

The cell classes belonging to the monocyte–macrophage lineage (mononuclear phagocyte system) are, in increasing order of maturity: monoblasts, promonocytes, marrow monocytes, blood monocytes and tissue macrophages.

Lymphocytopoiesis

The lymphoid stem cell in the bone marrow generates B-cell progenitors within that tissue. The B-cell progenitors undergo maturation into B cells in the microenvironment of the marrow and then travel via the blood into the B-cell zones of peripheral lymphoid tissue.

Either the lymphoid stem cells or primitive T-cell progenitors derived from them migrate from the marrow via the blood into the thymus where maturation into T cells takes place and those T cells which recognize self are deleted. The T cells later migrate to the T-cell zones of peripheral lymphoid organs.

The terms used to describe cells at various stages of B-lymphocyte differentiation in the bone marrow and T-lymphocyte differentiation in the thymus are as follows:

Early pre-B cell → pre-B cell → immature B cell → mature B cell
Thymic lymphoblast (prothymocyte) → stage I or early thymocyte → stage II or
    common thymocyte → stage III or mature thymocyte → mature T cell

All these stages have the morphological features of either lymphoblasts or lymphocytes. The identification of different lymphocyte precursors is therefore based not on morphology but on various properties like reactivity with certain monoclonal antibodies, immunoglobulin gene re-arrangement status, presence of immunoglobulin on the surface membrane, presence of μ-chains or immunoglobulin within the cytoplasm, terminal deoxynucleotidyl transferase activity and T-cell receptor gene rearrangement status.

Regulation of haemopoiesis

The regulation of haemopoietic stem cells seems to depend on intimate contact with one or more types of bone marrow stromal cell. The proliferation and maturation of committed progenitor cells are influenced by a number of haemopoietic growth factors secreted by stromal cells (macrophages, endothelial cells and fibroblasts). These include interleukin 3 (IL3), granulocyte–macrophage colony-stimulating factor (GM-CSF), granulocyte colony-stimulating factor (G-CSF) and macrophage colony-stimulating factor (M-CSF). The details of the steady-state regulation of blood cells other than red cells are still not entirely clear and will not be discussed further.

The rate of erythropoiesis is primarily regulated by the hormone erythropoietin which is secreted by the kidneys. The production of erythropoietin is stimulated when the supply of oxygen to renal tissue falls (i.e. when the red-cell count falls). Erythropoietin increases red-cell production mainly by stimulating the rate of conversion of CFU-E to pronormoblasts. It also shortens the total time taken for a pronormoblast to mature into marrow reticulocytes and for the latter to be released into the circulation.

BLOOD CELLS

Morphology

On Romanowsky-stained blood smears, normal erythrocytes appear as pink, anucleate cells with circular outlines and have diameters between 6.7 and 7.7

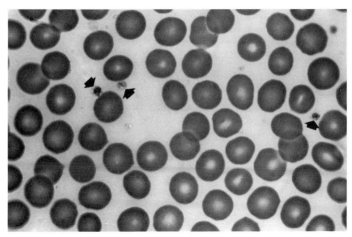

Fig. 1.6 Smear of normal peripheral venous blood. The red cells are round and do not vary greatly in size. They are well-filled with haemoglobin; the central area of pallor is small. A few platelets (arrowed) are also present.

μm (mean 7.2 μm). Blood-cell morphology should be assessed in a region of the blood smear in which only occasional red cells overlap. In such a region, each red cell (which is biconcave in shape) has a central area of pallor whose diameter is about a third of the red-cell diameter (Fig. 1.6).

In addition to red cells, blood smears contain platelets and various types of white cell. On average, the ratio between red cells, platelets and leucocytes is 700:40:1.

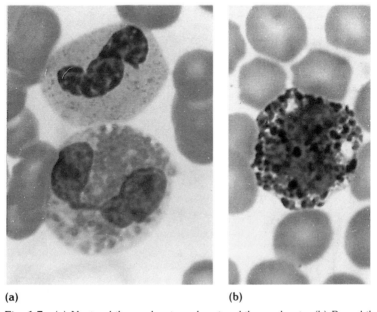

(a)   **(b)**

Fig. 1.7 (a) Neutrophil granulocyte and eosinophil granulocyte. (b) Basophil granulocyte.

The platelets are small anucleate cells, about 2–3 μm in diameter (Fig. 1.6). They stain light blue and contain a number of small azurophilic granules which are often concentrated at the centre. The important features of the morphology of normal leucocytes are summarized in Table 1.2. Neutrophil, eosinophil and basophil granulocytes (Fig. 1.7) are also described as polymorphonuclear leucocytes or polymorphs: the two or more nuclear masses in each cell are joined in series by fine strands of nuclear chromatin. Normally, the proportion of neutrophil polymorphs with five or more nuclear segments is 3% or less. Small lymphocytes (Fig. 1.8) account for about 90% of the lymphocytes in blood and large lymphocytes for the remaining 10%. Two monocytes from the peripheral blood of a normal adult are shown in Fig. 1.8.

Table 1.2 Morphology of normal white cells in Romanowsky-stained smears of peripheral blood.

Cell type	Cell size (μm)	Colour	Cytoplasm		Nucleus
			Ratio of cytoplasmic volume to nuclear volume	Granules	
Neutrophil granulocytes	9–15	Slightly pink	High	Numerous, very fine, faint purple	Usually 2–5 segments
Eosinophil granulocytes	12–17	Pale blue	High	Many, large and rounded, reddish-orange	Usually two segments
Basophil granulocytes	10–14		High	Several, large and rounded, dark purplish-black	Usually two segments, granules overlie nucleus
Monocytes	15–30	Pale greyish-blue, cytoplasmic vacuoles may be seen	Moderately high or high	Variable number, fine, purplish-red	Various shapes (rounded, C- or U-shaped, lobulated), skein-like or lacy chromatin
Lymphocytes	7–12 (small lymphocytes); 12–16 (large lymphocytes)	Pale blue	Low or very low	Few, fine, purplish-red	Rounded with large clumps of condensed chromatin

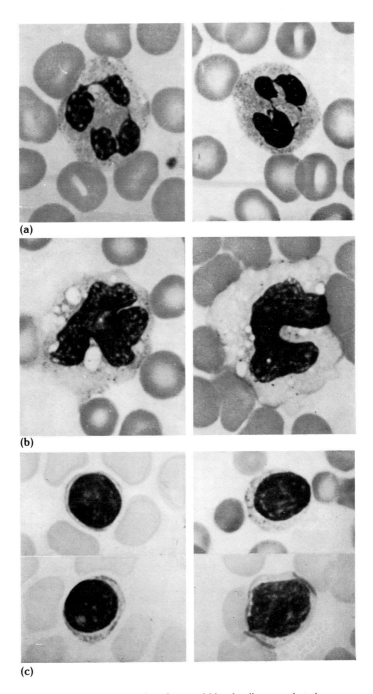

Fig. 1.8 Photomicrographs of normal blood cells printed at the same magnification. (a) Two neutrophil granulocytes. (b) Two monocytes. (c) Four lymphocytes of various sizes

Number and life-span

The normal ranges for the concentrations of various types of blood cell in adult Caucasians are given in Table 1.3, together with data on their life-span in the blood. Ranges for the Hb and PCV in healthy individuals are given on pp. 15–16. Normal red cells circulate for 110–120 days and at the end of their life-span are phagocytosed by cells of the mononuclear phagocyte system (reticuloendothelial system) in the bone marrow, spleen, liver and other organs.

The neutrophil granulocytes in the blood are distributed between a marginated granulocyte pool (consisting of cells that are loosely attached to the endothelial lining of small venules) and a circulating granulocyte pool. There is a continuous exchange of cells between these two pools and in healthy subjects, the circulating granulocyte pool accounts for between 16 and 99% (average, 44%) of all blood granulocytes. When cell counts are determined on samples of peripheral venous blood, only the circulating granulocytes are being studied. In healthy Caucasian adults, the normal range for the absolute neutrophil count is 1.5–7.5 $\times$ 10^9/litre. The lower limit for the normal range is lower in healthy Blacks, being about 1.0 $\times$ 10^9/litre. Neutrophil granulocytes leave the circulation exponentially, with an average $T_{1/2}$ of about 7 hours, and probably survive in tissues and secretions for about another 30 hours.

Lymphocytes continuously recirculate between the blood and the lymphatic system. They leave the blood between the endothelial cells of the post-capillary venules of lymph nodes, migrate through the lymph node into efferent lymphatics and re-enter the blood via the thoracic duct. The majority of human lymphocytes are long-lived, with average life-spans of 4–5 years and maximum life-spans greater than 20 years. The short-lived lymphocytes survive for about 3 days.

Table 1.3 Ninety five per cent confidence limits for the concentrations of various types of circulating blood cell in adult Caucasians and their life-span in the blood.

Cell type	Normal range (95% confidence limits)	Life-span in blood
Red cells	Males 4.4–5.8 $\times$ 10^{12}/litre Females 4.1–5.2 $\times$ 10^{12}/litre	110–120 days
White cells (leucocytes)	4.0–11.0 $\times$ 10^9/litre	
Neutrophil granulocytes	1.5–7.5 $\times$ 10^9/litre	$t_{1/2}$ approx. 7 hours
Eosinophil granulocytes	0.02–0.60 $\times$ 10^9/litre	$t_{1/2}$ approx. 6 hours
Basophil granulocytes	0.01–0.15 $\times$ 10^9/litre	
Monocytes	0.2–0.8 $\times$ 10^9/litre	$t_{1/2}$ approx. 70 hours
Lymphocytes	1.2–3.5 $\times$ 10^9/litre	
Platelets	160–450 $\times$ 10^9/litre	9–12 days

Functions

The main functions of blood cells are summarized in Table 1.4. More details of platelet function are given on pp. 162 and 163.

Lymphocytes

Between 65 and 80% of peripheral blood lymphocytes are T cells, 10–30% are B cells and 2–10% are non-T, non-B cells (null cells). Both B and T cells are formed with specific antigen-recognizing molecules on their cell surface which determine that each cell recognizes a specific antigenic determinant. The antigen-recognizing molecules for B and T cells are, respectively, immunoglobulin and the T-cell receptor molecule. The cells are triggered into proliferation when they react with the specific antigen in the presence of appropriate accessory cells, and their progeny develop into effector cells or memory cells.

The effector T-lymphocytes include helper cells (CD4-positive cells), which promote the function of B cells and are required for the maturation of other types of T cell, and suppressor-cytotoxic cells (CD8-positive cells) which inhibit the function of other lymphocytes and are cytotoxic towards foreign and virus-infected cells. The ratio of helper to suppressor cells is about 2:1. The null cells include killer (K) cells and natural killer (NK) cells. The killer cells lyse antibody-coated target cells and are therefore also called antibody-dependent cytotoxic cells (ADCC). The NK cells kill tumour cells and virus-infected cells in the absence of antibody. Thus, the functions of the T cells include:

1 mediation of cellular immunity against viruses, fungi and low-grade intracellular pathogens such as mycobacteria;

Table 1.4 Main functions of blood cells.

Type of cell	Main functions
Red blood cells (erythrocytes)	Transport O_2 from lungs to tissues; transport CO_2 from tissues to lungs
Granulocytes	
Neutrophil	Chemotaxis, phagocytosis, killing of phagocytosed bacteria
Eosinophil	All neutrophil functions listed above, effector cells for antibody-dependent damage to metazoal parasites, regulate immediate type hypersensitivity reactions (inactivate histamine and slow-reacting substance of anaphylaxis released by basophils and mast cells)
Basophil	Mediate immediate-type hypersensitivity (IgE-coated basophils react with specific antigen and release histamine and slow reacting substance of anaphylaxis), modulate inflammatory responses by releasing heparin and proteases
Monocytes	Chemotaxis, phagocytosis, killing of some microorganisms, become macrophages
Platelets	Adhere to subendothelial connective tissue, participate in blood clotting (see p. 162)
Lymphocytes	Involved in immune responses

2 participation in delayed hypersensitivity reactions, tumour rejection and graft rejection;

3 interaction with B cells in producing antibodies against certain antigens;

4 suppression of B-cell function.

T cells are also involved in the regulation of eosinophil granulocytopoiesis and, possibly, also of erythropoiesis.

The percentages of B cells that express IgM, IgD, IgG and IgA molecules on their surface are, respectively, 40, 30, 30 and 10. Many B cells have both IgM and IgD on their surface but others usually have only IgG or IgA. A single B cell expresses immunoglobulins of only one light chain type and there are twice as many cells with kappa light chains as there are with lambda light chains. B cells that are activated by reaction with specific antigen develop into antibody-secreting plasma cells or into B-memory cells. Most of the antibodies formed during a primary antibody response consist of IgM and almost all of the antibodies formed during a secondary antibody response (which results from the activation of B-memory cells) consist of IgG.

OBJECTIVES IN LEARNING

1 To understand the concept of a stem cell.

2 To understand where and how blood cells are produced from pluripotent haemopoietic stem cells and how erythropoiesis is regulated.

3 To be able to identify the various types of normal blood cell, erythroblasts and neutrophil precursors in colour transparencies.

4 To know the functions, concentration and life-span of various types of blood cell.

RECOMMENDED READING

Bessis M. (1973) *Living Blood Cells and their Ultrastructure.* Springer-Verlag, Berlin.

Potten CS (ed.) (1983) *Stem cells, their Identification and Characterisation.* Churchill Livingstone, Edinburgh.

Dunn CDR (ed.) (1983) *Current Concepts in Erythropoiesis.* John Wiley, Chichester.

Hardisty RM and Weatherall DJ (eds.) (1982) *Blood and its Disorders* (2nd edn). Blackwell Scientific Publications, Oxford.

Wickramasinghe SN (1975) *Human Bone Marrow.* Blackwell Scientific Publications, Oxford.

Wintrobe MM, Lee GR, Boggs DR, Bithell TC, Foerster J, Athens JW, Lukens JN. (1981) *Clinical Hematology* (8th edn). Lea & Febiger, Philadelphia,

Chapter 2
Anaemia and Polycythaemia: General Considerations

ANAEMIA

Anaemia is said to be present when the haemoglobin (Hb) concentration is below the normal range for the age and sex of an individual. Normal ranges for Hb concentration are given in Table 2.1. These are usually determined from a representative sample of healthy persons in whom the presence of nutritional deficiency has been excluded by specific laboratory investigations or by the prior administration of haematinics (e.g. iron). In populations with a high prevalence of α and β-thalassaemia genes, heterozygosity for thalassaemia may also have to be excluded. The average Hb level is 17.0 g/dl at birth and rises to 19.5 g/dl after 24 hours. Hb levels in children between 6 months and 6 years tend to be lower than in adults. The higher Hb levels in adult males than in adult non-pregnant females are largely due to the effects of higher androgen levels in males; the Hb levels of males fall after the age of 70 years. Hb levels are increased by residence at high altitude. Hb levels decrease during normal pregnancy, reaching their lowest value at about 32 weeks; the average fall is 1.5–2 g/dl. The drop in Hb concentration occurs despite an average increase in red cell mass of 300 ml, and results from an average increase in the plasma volume of about 1 litre. The Hb level may drop by 6–8% after 0.5 hours of bed rest.

Although normal ranges are invaluable in the assessment of a patient it must be realised that they do have some limitations. Thus, since normal ranges represent 95% confidence limits determined on a healthy population, it would be expected that 2.5% of healthy individuals have haemoglobin values below the normal range and that 2.5% have haemoglobin values above the normal range. Therefore, not all individuals with Hb levels slightly outside the normal range would necessarily have some haematological problem. Furthermore, as the difference between the upper and lower limits of the normal range is more than 3 g/dl, an individual's haemoglobin level may remain within the normal range even though it has fallen substantially due to some illness. In other words,

Table 2.1 Normal ranges for haemoglobin values.

	Hb concentration (g/dl)
Cord blood	13.5–20.5
First day of life	15.0–23.5
Children, 6 months–6 years	11.0–14.5
Children 6–14 years	12.0–15.5
Adult males	13.0–17.0
Adult females (non-pregnant)	12.0–15.5
Pregnant females	11.0–14.0

a 'normal' Hb concentration does not necessarily exclude impairment of erythropoiesis. It also does not exclude a moderate reduction in red cell life-span as the healthy bone marrow has a considerable physiological reserve and can increase the rate of effective erythropoiesis to 6–8 times the basal rate. The Hb level may be spuriously high in the presence of anaemia because of a decrease in the plasma volume secondary to dehydration.

In healthy individuals, there are strong correlations between the Hb, red cell count and packed cell volume (PCV). The normal ranges for the red-cell count in adult males and females are, respectively, $4.4–5.8 \times 10^{12}$/litre and $4.1–5.2 \times 10^{12}$/litre. The normal ranges for the PCV in adult males and females are 0.40–0.51 and 0.36–0.46, respectively.

Adaptive responses to anaemia

An important compensatory mechanism in anaemia consists of an increased production of 2,3-diphosphoglycerate (2,3-DPG) by red cells. This causes a reduction in the oxygen affinity of Hb (a shift of the oxygen dissociation curve to the right) and, consequently, increased release of oxygen at tissues. When the Hb falls below 7–8 g/dl, adaptive changes also occur in the cardiovascular system: these include an increase of cardiac output at rest mainly by an increase in stroke volume but also by an increase in heart rate.

Symptoms and signs of anaemia

Anaemia is a manifestation of disease, not a final diagnosis. The symptoms found in an anaemic patient may be caused by the underlying disease or by the anaemia itself. When anaemia develops slowly in children and young adults the symptoms referable to the anaemia are mild until the Hb falls below 7–8 g/dl. Significant symptoms develop at higher Hb levels in rapidly-developing anaemias and in older patients with impaired cardiovascular reserve. Older patients are also more likely to develop cardiac and cerebral symptoms than younger ones, due to associated degenerative vascular disease.

The two mechanisms underlying the many symptoms and signs of anaemia are:

1 decreased tissue oxygenation causing widespread organ dysfunction;
2 adaptive changes, particularly in the cardiovascular system.

Symptoms include lassitude, easy fatiguability, dyspnoea on exertion, palpitation, angina and intermittent claudication (in older patients with degenerative arterial disease), headache, vertigo, lightheadedness, visual disturbances, drowsiness, anorexia, nausea, bowel disturbances, menstrual disturbances, and loss of libido (see p. 69). Physical signs include pallor, tachycardia, wide pulse pressure with capillary pulsation, haemic murmurs, signs of congestive cardiac failure, and haemorrhages and occasional exudates in the retina. Severe anaemia may also cause slight proteinuria, mild impairment of renal function and low-grade fever.

Mechanisms of anaemia

In healthy adults, there is a steady-state equilibrium between the rate of release of new red cells from the bone marrow into the circulation and the rate of removal of senescent red cells from the circulation by the mononuclear

Table 2.2   Mechanisms of anaemia.

Blood loss

Decreased red cell life-span (haemolytic anaemia)
  Congenital defect (e.g. sickle-cell disease, hereditary spherocytosis)
  Acquired defect (e.g. malaria, some drugs)

Impairment of red cell formation
  Abnormality of Hb synthesis
  Abnormality of other erythroblast functions (e.g. abnormal cell proliferation)

Pooling and destruction of red cells in an enlarged spleen

Increased plasma volume (splenomegaly, pregnancy)

phagocyte system. The various mechanisms which may lead to anaemia are shown in Table 2.2. More than one of these mechanisms operate simultaneously in most conditions, and mechanistic classifications of the anaemias have to be based on the mechanism of greatest pathophysiological importance.

Blood loss

The loss of 500 ml of blood over a few minutes usually has negligible effects on the circulatory system; there is a slight fall in central venous pressure and no significant change in blood pressure or pulse rate. The rapid loss of 750 ml causes a substantial fall in central venous pressure, a fall in cardiac output and blood pressure and peripheral vasoconstriction. The acute loss of 1.5–2 litres of blood causes marked circulatory disturbances: the subjects are cold, clammy and restless and may become unconscious.

Immediately after an acute haemorrhage, the haemoglobin level is normal. The acute reduction in blood volume is corrected by a slow expansion of the plasma volume over the next 36–72 hours. This results in the gradual development of a normochromic normocytic anaemia, with the lowest haemoglobin values between 36 and 72 hours. Other changes seen in the blood after acute haemorrhage include:

1   reticulocytosis (with a peak at 7–10 days);
2   moderate neutrophil leucocytosis and mild thrombocytosis lasting for several days;
3   the presence of metamyelocytes and occasional myelocytes in the blood film. Normoblasts may appear in the blood after severe haemorrhage.

Chronic blood loss eventually causes a hypochromic microcytic anaemia due to iron deficiency.

Other mechanisms

The anaemias resulting partly or wholly from a substantial reduction of red cell life-span are discussed in Chapter 3. The diseases associated with impaired red-cell formation are listed in Table 2.3. In chronic renal failure, anaemia is mainly caused by decreased erythropoietin production in the diseased kidneys and by the inhibitory effects of 'uraemic toxins' on the marrow.

Table 2.3 Causes of impaired red cell formation.

Deficiency of essential haematinics
    Iron, folate, vitamin B_{12}, protein, vitamin C

Chronic disorders
    Infection, renal disease, liver disease, collagen disease

Marrow infiltration
    Carcinoma, myeloma, leukaemia, lymphoma,
    myelofibrosis, lipid storage diseases (e.g.
    Gaucher's disease), marble bone disease

Endocrine deficiency
    Hypofunction of the thyroid, testes, adrenal
    glands or anterior lobe of the pituitary gland

Myelotoxic agents, aplastic anaemia and pure red cell aplasia

Miscellaneous
    Vitamin B_{12}-independent and folate-independent
    megaloblastic anaemias, β-thalassaemia syndromes,
    myelodysplastic syndromes (including primary acquired
    sideroblastic anaemia), congenital dyserythropoietic
    anaemias, malaria

Morphological classification of anaemia

A useful method for classifying anaemias is based on the morphology of red cells in a stained blood smear. The main terms used in such a classification are normocytic, microcytic, macrocytic, normochromic and hypochromic. *Normocytes* are red cells with a normal diameter; *microcytes* and *macrocytes* are those with a reduced and increased diameter, respectively (Figs. 2.1 a–c). *Normochromia* implies normal staining of the cell, with the central area of pallor occupying about a third of the cell diameter (Fig. 2.1a) and *hypochromia* indicates reduced staining, with an increase in the central area of pallor (Fig. 2.1b). Today, morphological classification is based not only on morphological criteria but also on mean cell volume (MCV) values determined by automated blood-counting machines. It must be appreciated, however, that when blood contains a small proportion of microcytes or macrocytes, the MCV is within the normal range. The three morphological types of anaemia and examples of conditions causing them are given in Table 2.4. The normal values for the MCV and other red cell indices in adults are given in Table 2.5.

There are a number of morphological abnormalities of red cells other than those just mentioned which may be seen on a stained blood film in a patient with anaemia; some of these are mentioned below.

Anisocytosis and poikilocytosis

An increased degree of variation in cell diameter (anisocytosis) or cell shape (poikilocytosis) may be seen in many conditions associated with disturbed erythropoiesis. They are not specific for any disease.

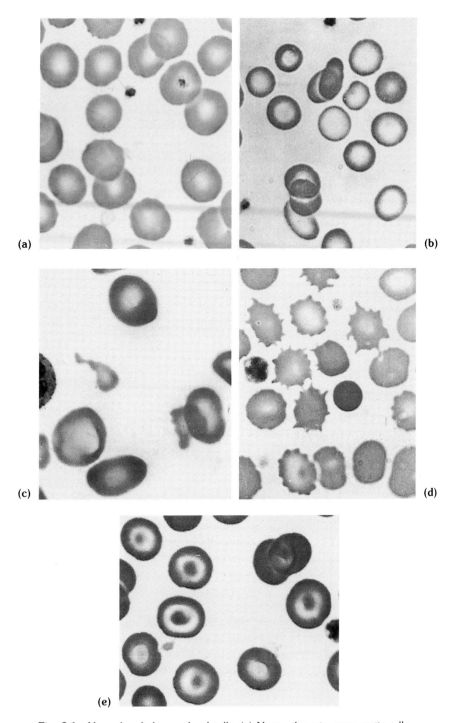

Fig. 2.1 Normal and abnormal red cells. (a) Normochromic, normocytic cells. (b) Hypochromic microcytic cells. (c) Macrocytes and two poikilocytes. (d) One spherocyte and several acanthocytes in a blood-film from a splenectomized patient. Acanthocytes are red cells with up to about 10 spicules of varying length irregularly distributed over their surface. They are found not only post-splenectomy but also in other conditions such as hypothyroidism and advanced alcohol-related cirrhosis of the liver. (e) Target cells from a patient with obstructive jaundice.

Table 2.4 Morphological classification of anaemia.

Type	MCV	Causes
Microcytic and hypochromic, or microcytic*	Low	Iron deficiency, thalassaemia syndromes, some cases of anaemia of chronic disorders
Normocytic and normochromic	Normal	Acute blood loss, some cases of anaemia of chronic disorders, some haemolytic anaemias, leucoerythroblastic anaemias
Macrocytic	High	Alcoholism, folate deficiency, vitamin B_{12} deficiency (see Chapter 6 for other causes)

*Microcytic red cells do not always appear hypochromic on a blood film.

Table 2.5 Normal values for red cell indices in adults.

Index	Normal range
Mean cell volume (MCV)*	82–99 fl
Mean cell haemogloblin (MCH)	27–33 pg
Mean cell haemoglobin concentration (MCHC)	32–36 g/dl

*Lower limit may be as low as 70–74 fl between 1 and 8 years of age, in the absence of iron deficiency.

Target cells

These are abnormally thin red cells which have well-stained areas in their middle and periphery and a pale area in between (Fig. 2.1e); they are found in thalassaemia syndromes, iron deficiency, sickle-cell anaemia, heterozygotes and homozygotes for haemoglobin C, homozygotes for haemoglobin E, liver disease, obstructive jaundice, hyposplenism and splenectomized individuals.

Spherocytes or microspherocytes

In several different types of haemolytic anaemia, some red cells lose their biconcave shape and become more-or-less spherical. In blood films, they appear as deeply-stained cells which have lost their central area of pallor and which have smaller diameters than normal cells (Fig. 2.1d). Spherocytes are classically found in hereditary spherocytosis and in autoimmune haemolytic anaemias with warm reactive antibodies. They are also found when red cells are damaged by heat (as in patients with burns) and by various chemicals.

Howell–Jolly bodies (Fig. 2.2)

These small rounded intraerythrocytic inclusions consist of nuclear material. They are found in circulating red cells following splenectomy or in patients with

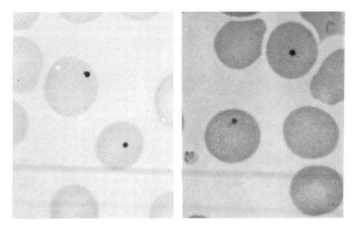

Fig. 2.2   Peripheral blood smear from a splenectomized patient with hereditary spherocytosis showing Howell–Jolly bodies within four of the red cells.

hyposplenism. Howell–Jolly bodies are normally present in some red cells when they leave the marrow but are rapidly removed by the spleen, possibly during the first passage of the inclusion-containing cells through that organ; consequently, they are not found in blood films of individuals with a functioning spleen. In megaloblastic anaemias, the formation of Howell–Jolly bodies within the erythroblasts in the marrow is greatly increased and when megaloblastic haemopoiesis is associated with splenectomy or hyposplenism, the peripheral blood contains very large numbers of red cells with these inclusions.

POLYCYTHAEMIA (ERYTHROCYTOSIS)

The term polycythaemia is usually applied when the packed cell volume (PCV) is repeatedly greater than 0.52 in adult males and 0.47 in adult females in peripheral blood samples taken without venous occlusion. The increase in PCV is associated with a high Hb level and a high red-cell count. Polycythaemia may result either from an increase in the total volume of red cells in the circulation (true polycythaemia) or from a decrease in the total plasma volume (apparent or relative polycythaemia). Thus, measurements of total red-cell volume (using ^{51}Cr- or ^{99m}Tc-labelled red cells) and plasma volume (using ^{125}I-albumin) are often required in the investigation of patients. The total red-cell volume (red-cell mass) is expressed as a percentage of the value predicted for the height and weight of the individual being studied; the predicted value is obtained using formulae which take some account of the amount of relatively avascular fatty tissue in the body. A patient is considered to have true polycythaemia when the measured total red-cell volume exceeds the predicted value by more than 25% in males and 30% in females. The disorders associated with true and apparent polycythaemia are given in Table 2.6.

An important cause of true polycythaemia, namely polycythaemia rubra vera, is discussed on p. 131. In most of the conditions listed as causing inappropriate erythropoietin production in Table 2.6, the high erythropoietin levels are either secreted by tumour cells or by compressed and hypoxic normal

Table 2.6   Causes of polycythaemia.

True polycythaemia	Apparent polycythaemia (relative polycythaemia)

Primary
  Polycythaemia rubra vera (p. 131),
  Idiopathic erythrocytosis (p. 134)
	Dehydration
	  Vomiting
	  diarrhoea
	  burns
	  inadequate fluid intake

Secondary
Due to generalized tissue hypoxia causing
appropriately increased erythropoietin production
  High altitude, cyanotic heart disease, chronic
  hypoxic pulmonary disease, alveolar
  hypoventilation due to gross obesity, heavy
  smoking (formation of carboxyhaemoglobin),
  abnormal haemoglobin with high oxygen affinity
  (e.g. Hb Chesapeake)
	Stress polycythaemia
	  (Also called spurious polycythaemia or
	  Gaisböck's syndrome)

Due to inappropriately increased erythropoietin
production
  Kidney disease (carcinoma, cysts, hydronephrosis),
  renal transplantation, hepatocellular carcinoma,
  cerebellar haemangioblastoma, massive uterine
  fibromyomata	

renal tissue surrounding renal cysts or tumours. Occasionally, there may be increased production of erythropoietin in the absence of generalized hypoxia due to an impairment of renal blood flow causing selective renal hypoxia. From the many causes of secondary polycythaemia shown in the table, it is evident that the diagnosis of the cause of a true polycythaemia may require a number of investigations such as the measurement of the oxygen saturation of arterial blood, haemoglobin electrophoresis (which detects two-thirds of the abnormal haemoglobins with a high oxygen affinity), determination of haemoglobin oxygen dissociation curves, intravenous pyelography, and measurement of serum erythropoietin levels.

Chronic apparent polycythaemia (stress polycythaemia) is a condition of unknown aetiology which is usually seen in middle-aged, obese individuals who tend to be anxious. Affected individuals are often hypertensive.

Polycythaemia due to any cause is accompanied by an increase in whole blood viscosity. When symptoms are present, they are generally attributed to a decrease in blood flow through the limbs, heart and brain as a consequence of the increased viscosity. In polycythaemia rubra vera, there is a high incidence of vaso-occlusive episodes related partly to the hyperviscosity and partly to a high platelet count. The risk of vaso-occlusive episodes in secondary polycythaemia has not yet been adequately documented and may be considerably less than in polycythaemia rubra vera. However, thrombotic episodes have been reported in occasional patients with polycythaemia secondary to cyanotic heart disease and high-affinity haemoglobins. Although patients with stress polycythaemia are undoubtedly prone to suffer from coronary artery thrombosis and cerebrovascular accidents, the role of the high PCV in the pathogenesis of the vascular disease and vaso-occlusive episodes is still unclear.

Whereas venesection has a clear role in the management of polycythaemia rubra vera (p. 134), its role in the management of secondary polycythaemia and stress polycythaemia remains uncertain. Some physicians cautiously venesect only those patients with symptoms attributable to hyperviscosity or with symptoms from coronary artery or cerebrovascular insufficiency; in secondary polycythaemia, the PCV should not be reduced to less than 0.50–0.52 since the polycythaemia has developed to compensate for poor oxygen delivery to tissues. In polycythaemia secondary to hypoxic pulmonary disease, venesection has been shown to improve cardiac function and cerebral blood flow.

OBJECTIVES IN LEARNING

1   To know how the symptoms and signs of anaemia and polycythaemia are caused.

2   To understand the mechanisms and the morphological classification of anaemia.

3   To know the causes of true and apparent polycythaemia.

Chapter 3
Haemolytic Anaemias

Under the heading of haemolytic anaemias are grouped a number of diseases which have one abnormality in common, namely, a shortened red cell life-span. It should be noted that a patient with a diminished red cell life-span is not always anaemic. When patients have only a moderate reduction in red cell life-span, say 30 days instead of the normal 120 days, they are capable of increasing the rate of red-cell production to maintain the haemoglobin concentration within normal limits, provided that their bone marrow is healthy. Such individuals are described as suffering from a compensated haemolytic state rather than a haemolytic anaemia. In the majority of haemolytic anaemias, the cells of the reticuloendo-thelial system in the spleen, liver and bone marrow remove the abnormal red cells from the circulation by phagocytosis (extravascular haemolysis). In a minority, the red cells rupture and release their haemoglobin intravascularly (intravascular haemolysis).

Haemolytic anaemias are uncommon diseases amongst the indigenous population of the UK. However, in the multiracial communities now found in and around London and some other major cities, patients with haemolytic anaemias are encountered more frequently. There are a considerable number of diseases which are associated with a haemolytic process. The student need only be familiar with those diseases which are most commonly encountered. These include: hereditary spherocytosis, hereditary elliptocytosis, glucose-6-phosphate dehydrogenase deficiency, sickle-cell anaemia, thalassaemia and the acquired haemolytic anaemias. Those who wish to learn about other haemolytic diseases should consult the monographs of Dacie (1967, 1985 and 1988).

EVIDENCE OF HAEMOLYSIS

When the rate of red-cell destruction is increased, red-cell production in the marrow is stimulated through the erythropoietin mechanism in an attempt to maintain the haemoglobin concentration at the normal level. In the majority of haemolytic anaemias, the marrow responds optimally to this stimulus and increases the red-cell output up to a maximum of 6–8 times normal. However, a suboptimal marrow response is seen when there is a lack of iron, B_{12} or folic acid or when the red-cell precursors are damaged (sometimes by the agent causing the haemolysis) or when the marrow is infiltrated by malignant cells (e.g. in chronic lymphocytic leukaemia complicated by an autoimmune haemolytic anaemia). Since haemolysis is usually associated with increased erythropoiesis, two categories of laboratory evidence can be looked for in a patient suspected of suffering from a haemolytic state. These are: (a) evidence of increased red-cell destruction; and (b) evidence of a compensatory increase in erythropoietic activity.

Laboratory evidence of increased red-cell destruction

The various types of evidence in this category are summarized in Table 3.1.

Biochemical consequences of extravascular haemolysis

The simplest method of obtaining evidence of increased red-cell destruction is by estimating the amount of bilirubin and its derivatives in plasma, faeces and urine. When the red cell is destroyed within macrophages, the haem is converted into bilirubin with the release of carbon monoxide. Free bilirubin is insoluble in water and hence is transported to the liver attached to albumin. In the liver it is converted into the soluble glucuronide and excreted. The healthy liver is capable of handling more bilirubin than is normally produced and is able to increase its bilirubin-handling capacity further in haemolytic states. However, there is an upper limit for the rate of glucuronide formation by the liver and when the supply of bilirubin exceeds this rate, the bilirubin concentration in the plasma rises. Bilirubin concentration therefore does not rise above the normal range when there is only a moderate increase in the rate of destruction of red cells. It begins to rise when the life-span is shortened to about 50 days or less. A rise in plasma bilirubin concentration is only significant in the diagnosis of a haemolytic process if liver function is entirely normal.

As far as is known, bilirubin is not catabolized in the body, but excreted in the faeces where it is converted by bacteria into urobilinogen. As an average-sized adult destroys about 20 ml of red cells each day, this should result in the excretion of 200 mg of urobilinogen. When there is an excessive rate of destruction of red cells, the amount of urobilinogen in the faeces rises and causes the faeces to be darker than normal. Estimation of the amount of urobilinogen excreted in the faeces can be used to obtain evidence of a haemolytic process, but is now rarely carried out, since the diagnosis can usually be substantiated by other tests.

Table 3.1 Laboratory findings indicative of increased red cell destruction.

Biochemical consequences of extravascular haemolysis
Hyperbilirubinaemia (unconjugated)
Increased urinary urobilinogen
Increased faecal urobilinogen
Reduced serum haptoglobin
Biochemical consequences of intravascular haemolysis
Reduced serum haptoglobin
Haemoglobinaemia
Methaemalbuminaemia
Reduced haemopexin levels
Haemoglobinuria
Haemosiderinuria
Morphological evidence of damage to red cells
Microspherocytes, red-cell fragments, sickle cells
Reduced red cell life-span

Some urobilinogen is always reabsorbed from the gut and excreted in the urine. When the concentration in the faeces increases, the amount excreted in the urine also increases, and this can be detected with Ehrlich's aldehyde reagent.

Biochemical consequences of intravascular haemolysis

The haemoglobin released from intravascular lysis of red cells binds to the specific haemoglobin-binding protein in the plasma, namely haptoglobin. Since the haemoglobin–haptoglobin complexes are rapidly taken up by cells of the mononuclear phagocyte system, intravascular haemolysis leads to a reduction in haptoglobin levels. Haptoglobins may also be reduced in extravascular haemolysis, due to the escape of some haemoglobin from the macrophages which phagocytose damaged red cells.

When the quantity of haemoglobin released during intravascular haemolysis exceeds the haemoglobin-binding capacity of haptoglobin, free haemoglobin is found in the plasma (haemoglobinaemia). Haem is released from the haemoglobin and rapidly becomes oxidized to haematin. The oxidized haem initially binds to the specific haem-binding protein in plasma, haemopexin; the haem-haemopexin complexes are cleared by hepatocytes. After the haemopexin molecules are saturated, the haematin binds to albumin, to form methaemalbumin which can be detected by the Schumm's test. When haemoglobinaemia is present, some of the free haemoglobin dissociates into dimers and the dimers pass through the glomerulus, thus causing haemoglobinuria. Some of the dimers are taken up by renal tubular cells and deposited within the cells as haemosiderin. The haemosiderin may be detected in spun deposits of urine both inside shed tubular cells and extracellularly, using Perls' acid ferrocyanide reaction.

Morphological evidence of damage to red cells

A careful examination of a blood film may indicate the occurence of haemolysis by revealing the presence of damaged or abnormal red cells such as microspherocytes, schistocytes (red-cell fragments), sickled red cells or cells containing malarial parasites.

Reduced red cell life-span

The best way to show that the red cell life-span is shortened is to label the red cells with radioactive chromium (^{51}Cr) and reinject them into the patient (Mollison et al.1987). The survival of the labelled cells can then be followed by taking blood samples at suitable intervals and measuring their radioactivity. The analysis of the survival curve is complicated by the fact that the ^{51}Cr slowly elutes out of the red cells at a constant rate, but a correction can be made for this. The use of ^{51}Cr as a red-cell label has the advantage that an indication of the main site of red-cell destruction can be obtained. ^{51}Cr emits γ-rays which will penetrate the body tissue and thus ^{51}Cr deposited in the spleen or liver can be detected by placing a γ-ray detector on the surface of the body over these organs. Experience has shown that when the ^{51}Cr accumulates predominantly in the spleen in haemolytic anaemias, splenectomy is usually followed by a partial or complete cure of the haemolytic process (Fig. 3.1).

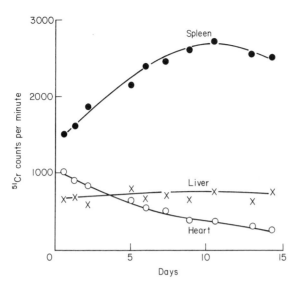

Fig. 3.1 The excessive accumulation of ^{51}Cr in the spleen (•) compared to the liver (x) and heart (○) in a patient with idiopathic autoimmune haemolytic anaemia. In this patient, splenectomy was followed by a complete remission. ^{51}Cr counts obtained over the spleen in normal people are similar to counts over the liver.

The extent of the shortening of the red cell life-span in disease varies according to the type of disease and also between different individuals with the same disease. For example, in those patients with hereditary spherocytosis who have no anaemia, red-cell survival may only be shortened to 30 days, a value well within the ability of the marrow to compensate (Fig. 3.2). On the other hand, a life-span as short as 5 days, irrespective of its cause, is always associated with severe anaemia.

Laboratory evidence of increased erythropoietic activity

If evidence can be obtained of an increased rate of red-cell production, this suggests that a haemolytic process is taking place, providing that there has been no loss of red cells through haemorrhage and the patient is not responding to therapy with iron, vitamin B$_{12}$ or folate. Two simple measurements can be used for assessing whether there is any increase in the rate of formation of red cells, namely, the reticulocyte count in the peripheral blood and the myeloid/erythroid ratio in the marrow (Table 3.2).

Reticulocytosis (increased reticulocyte count)

The number of reticulocytes in the peripheral blood is expressed either as a percentage of the total number of red cells or as an absolute number per litre of blood; in normal adults, the percentage is in the range of 0.8–3.7% and the absolute count is $18–158 \times 10^9$/litre. In theory, the total number of reticulocytes in the circulation should be proportional to the rate of production of red cells, provided that there is no variation in the length of time that reticulocytes

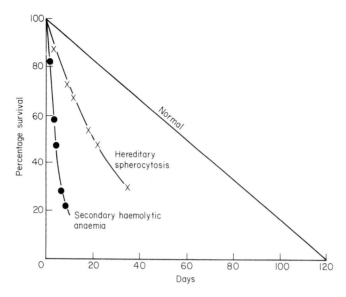

Fig. 3.2   The survival of ^{51}Cr-labelled red cells (corrected for ^{51}Cr elution) in the circulation of: a patient with hereditary spherocytosis (x) whose haemoglobin concentration was 15.5 g/dl, the mean red cell life-span 30 days; and a patient with autoimmune haemolytic anaemia secondary to chronic lymphocytic leukaemia (•), whose haemoglobin concentration was 5 g/dl; the mean red cell life-span 5 days.

take to mature. In practice, reticulocytes released prematurely from the marrow following erythropoietin stimulation do spend longer in the circulation before they mature into adult cells. Nevertheless, an increase in the absolute reticulocyte count is an indication of increased erythropoietic activity and in general, the higher the count, the greater the rate of delivery of viable red cells to the circulation. The reticulocyte percentage may increase up to 50% or more when erythropoietic activity is intense.

Erythroblastaemia and macrocytosis

Moderate or marked erythroid hyperplasia may be associated with the presence of occasional nucleated red cells (erythroblasts) in the circulation (erythroblastaemia). A high mean cell volume (MCV) that is unrelated to folate deficiency may also occur. This macrocytosis is related to the presence of a high proportion

Table 3.2   Evidence of increased erythropoietic activity.

Peripheral blood
    Reticulocytosis and erythroblastaemia; macrocytosis

Bone marrow
    Erythroid hyperplasia; reduced
    myeloid/erythroid ratio

Bone
    Changes in the skull and tubular bones

of reticulocytes in the blood and to the fact that the reticulocytes formed during accelerated erythropoiesis are abnormally large and mature into rounded macrocytes. Erythroid hyperplasia also imposes an increased demand for folate and if this is not met by adequate dietary intake, macrocytosis due to folate deficiency develops.

Erythroid hyperplasia and reduced myeloid/erythroid (M/E) ratio

A semi-quantitative assessment of the degree of erythroid hyperplasia can be obtained by determining the M/E ratio in the bone marrow. This is often defined as the ratio between the number of cells of the neutrophil series (including mature granulocytes) and the number of erythroblasts in bone marrow. The normal range for the M/E ratio in marrow smears from adults is 2.0–8.3 (i.e. there are normally more cells of the neutrophil series than erythroblasts). A reduction of the M/E ratio is taken as evidence of erythroid hyperplasia, provided that the total number of cells of the neutrophil series can be assumed to be normal. Marrows showing erythroid hyperplasia are hypercellular, due to the replacement of fat cells by erythroblasts (Plates 5–7). When erythroid hyperplasia is marked, fat cells may be virtually absent. Also, haemopoietic tissue may extend into marrow cavities which usually contain only fat, and extramedullary haemopoiesis may develop in the liver, spleen and lymph nodes.

Erythroid hyperplasia occurs not only in haemolytic states and after haemorrhage but also in megaloblastic and sideroblastic anaemias (where erythropoiesis is markedly ineffective, see p. 5), polycythaemia and erythroleukaemia.

Clinical features of haemolytic states

These result both from the increased red-cell destruction and from the compensatory increase in erythropoietic activity. There may be pallor and mild jaundice. The prevalence of pigment stones in the gall bladder is increased; the stones may occasionally cause deep jaundice due to biliary obstruction. Splenomegaly is common. In patients with severe congenital haemolytic anaemias, the erythroid hyperplasia causes expansion of marrow cavities, thinning of cortical bone, bone deformities (e.g. frontal and parietal bossing) and, very occasionally, pathological fractures. These changes cause characteristic radiological abnormalities in the skull and other bones (Fig. 3.3). Occasionally, chronic leg ulcers develop over the malleoli.

Aplastic crises

Episodes of pure red-cell aplasia, lasting about 1 week, may complicate the course of patients with chronic haemolytic anaemia. Erythroblasts virtually disappear from the marrow, the absolute reticulocyte count falls markedly (sometimes to zero) and the haemoglobin falls rapidly. Such crises are usually due to infection by a parvovirus. Affected patients may have to be transfused with red cells urgently.

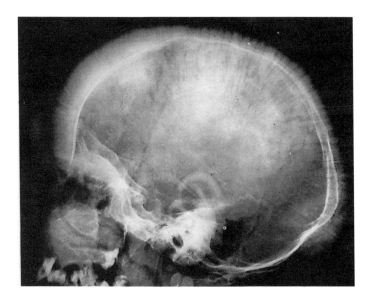

Fig. 3.3 X-ray of the skull of a patient with sickle-cell anaemia. The space between the two abnormally thin tables of the frontal and parietal bones is considerably widened due to erythroid hyperplasia. Bone trabeculae have developed at right angles to the tables giving a 'hair-on-end' appearance.

DIAGNOSIS OF HAEMOLYTIC ANAEMIA

There are two stages in the diagnosis:

1 the demonstration of a haemolytic state;

2 the determination of its aetiology.

The diagnosis of a haemolytic state is commonly made with reasonable confidence by the finding of an increase in both the reticulocyte count and the plasma bilirubin concentration, in a patient in whom alternative causes for the latter two abnormalities are excluded, e.g. haemorrhage and liver disease. Anaemia may or may not be present. Other findings indicating haemolysis have been discussed above (see Tables 3.1 and 3.2).

The next stage in diagnosis is to determine the nature of the disease which is causing the haemolysis. In approaching the diagnosis, it is useful to make a distinction between congenital abnormalities of the red cells on the one hand, and acquired abnormalities on the other. In the latter category, an agent acts on the red cell leading to its destruction, e.g. autoantibodies in autoimmune haemolytic anaemia. Congenital haemolytic anaemias may result from defects in one of three components of the red cell:

1 cell membrane;

2 enzyme systems concerned with the energy production that maintains the integrity of the cell;

3 haemoglobin.

CONGENITAL HAEMOLYTIC ANAEMIAS

Defects of the red cell membrane

There is a filamentous protein meshwork which is attached to the inner surface of the red cell membrane, called the membrane cytoskeleton. The four main proteins in this cytoskeleton are spectrin, actin, protein 4.1 and ankyrin. The cytoskeleton seems to be important for maintaining the normal biconcave shape of the red cell.

Hereditary spherocytosis

The most common example of a haemolytic anaemia due to a membrane defect is hereditary spherocytosis (HS). Recent evidence indicates that there is a reduction in the spectrin content of erythrocytes in many patients and defective interaction between spectrin and protein 4.1 in others (Agre *et al.* 1986). The abnormality appears to cause the older red cells to become microspherocytes. Repeated passage through the spleen aggravates the spherocytic change. Spherocytes are less deformable than normal red cells and are therefore retarded and eventually prevented from passing from the Billroth cords to the splenic sinusoids. The trapped cells are engulfed and destroyed by splenic macrophages, thus leading to a reduction in red-cell survival.

The prevalence of the disease in North Europe has been estimated to be 2–3 per 10 000 of the population, so that a large general practice in London may contain one family with the disease (Mackinney 1965). The disease is usually inherited as an autosomal dominant character. Patients often give a family history of the condition, such as a parent or sibling who is known to have the disease or who has had recurrent anaemia, gall stones or a splenectomy.

The disease may present at any time from birth to old-age, although it is usually the mildly affected patients who reach adulthood without detection. There is a great difference in the severity of the disease, varying from patients who have a haemoglobin concentration of 4–5 g/dl to patients who are not anaemic at all and who are only diagnosed during a routine examination of a blood film or who may present because they have a family history of the disease and desire investigation. Mackinney (1965) investigated 26 families and found that half the patients had no symptoms but had abnormal findings in the peripheral blood. He also found that half the non-splenectomized patients had haemoglobin concentrations of over 12 g/dl.

Apart from anaemia and jaundice, the main clinical finding in most patients is an enlarged spleen, although this may not be palpable in a mild case. Most patients develop pigment stones in the gall bladder, but only 10–20% of those with intact spleens develop acute cholecystitis or biliary obstruction.

The rate of destruction of red cells in a particular patient remains fairly constant but episodes of increased destruction may occur during which the patient becomes more jaundiced and more anaemic and frequently develops abdominal pain. Aplastic or hypoplastic crises due to a temporary failure of red-cell production by the bone marrow may also occur and are characterized by a rapid and marked fall in the reticulocyte count and haemoglobin concentration. These hypoplastic or aplastic crises are often preceded by a trivial febrile illness such as an upper respiratory tract infection, and seem to be caused by infection of erythroid progenitor cells with parvovirus B19. Patients may present for the first time during a haemolytic or aplastic episode.

Megaloblastic anaemia due to folate deficiency may also be found, as in other chronic haemolytic disorders. This results from an increased requirement for folate by the hyperactive bone marrow, and is especially found when the diet is inadequate.

Diagnosis

The cardinal clinical features are a family history, mild jaundice, pallor and splenomegaly. The laboratory findings which are of the greatest help in diagnosis are: the presence of spherocytes in the stained blood-film (Fig. 3.4), an increased reticulocyte count, raised plasma bilirubin, increased osmotic fragility of the red cells, a negative antiglobulin test (which excludes spherocytosis due to an autoantibody) and anaemia. Only a small percentage of the red cells are spherocytes and they appear as small densely staining cells. An important test which must always be carried out is the osmotic fragility test. When normal red cells are suspended in a range of hypotonic saline solutions, they do not start to lyse until the saline concentration is reduced below 0.55 g/dl. In hereditary spherocytosis, the red cells are thicker than normal and some are already spherocytic, so that a fluid uptake smaller than normal is sufficient to burst the cells (i.e. the cells have an increased osmotic fragility). Thus, these abnormal cells start to lyse when the saline concentration is as high as 0.6–0.8 g/dl.

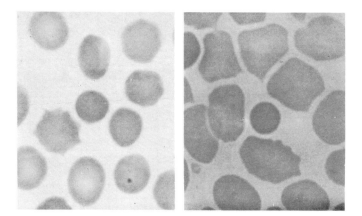

Fig. 3.4 Blood film from a patient with hereditary spherocytosis. There is one spherocyte in the centre of each photograph.

Treatment

It is usual to subject all patients other than those who are mildly affected to splenectomy. Since splenectomy, particularly in children under the age of 5 years, is associated with an increased risk of fatal infections, it should be delayed until after the age of 5–10 years, whenever possible. Splenectomy regularly results in a rise in the haemoglobin level, the disappearance of jaundice and an increase of red cell life-span to almost normal values. However, spherocytosis persists.

Hereditary elliptocytosis

This condition, which affects 4 per 10 000 of the population, is transmitted as an autosomal dominant trait. Characteristically, 25–90% of the red cells are oval, elliptical or rod-shaped (Fig. 3.5). Most heterozygotes are not anaemic and some show evidence of a compensated haemolytic state. Homozygotes usually have a severe haemolytic anaemia from infancy. The primary defect is an abnormality in the membrane cytoskeleton. Many patients have various mutations affecting spectrin or protein 4.1 and some lack protein 4.1 (Palek 1985).

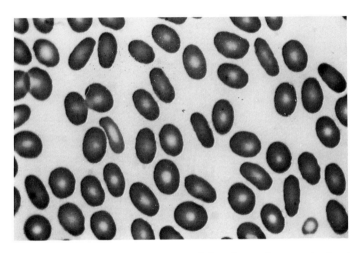

Fig. 3.5 Blood film from a patient with hereditary elliptocytosis showing a high proportion of elliptical red cells.

Abnormalities of red-cell enzymes

Haemolytic anaemias may also result from congenital abnormalities of the enzyme system concerned with energy transfer in glucose metabolism (Mentzer 1981). The red cell requires a continuous supply of energy for the maintenance of membrane flexibility and cell shape, the regulation of the sodium and potassium pumps, and the maintenance of haemoglobin in the reduced ferrous form. The energy is obtained from glucose which is converted to lactic acid mainly through the anaerobic glycolytic cycle (Embden–Meyerhof pathway). There is an alternative aerobic pathway, the pentose-phosphate shunt, starting with glucose-6-phosphate and requiring glucose-6-phosphate dehydrogenase (G6PD) as the initial enzyme (Fig. 3.6). Energy is transferred through the energy-rich compounds adenosine triphosphate (ATP), reduced nicotinamide-adenine dinucleotide (NADH), the related phosphorylated compound, NADPH, and reduced glutathione (GSH).

The discovery that congenital deficiences of some of the enzymes concerned with glucose metabolism give rise to haemolytic anaemia is fairly recent. It was

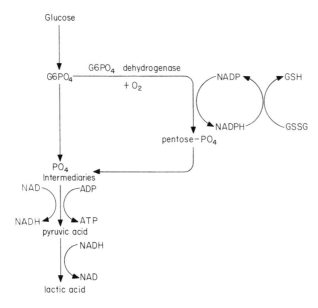

Fig. 3.6   A schematic diagram of the pathway of glucose metabolism in the red cell, to show the important role of glucose-6-PO$_4$ dehydrogenase. Decreased activity of the enzyme leads to a deficiency of the reducing compounds NADPH and GSH.

noticed in the decade 1920–30 that the antimalarial drugs, aminoquinolines, produced a haemolytic anaemia in certain Black individuals, but it was not until the work of Beutler (1959) that this was found to be due to a congenital deficiency of glucose-6-phosphate dehydrogenase. At about the same time, it was also noticed that there was a type of congenital haemolytic anaemia which could be distinguished from hereditary spherocytosis by the absence of sphero-cytes and the failure to respond to splenectomy (Haden 1947); it was termed congenital non-spherocytic haemolytic anaemia. It is now known that many of these latter patients have enzyme deficiencies within the pentose–phosphate shunt or the glycolytic cycle, most commonly of G6PD and occasionally of other enzymes such as pyruvate kinase. The most prevalent G6PD enzyme with normal activity world-wide is designated type B.

Glucose-6-phosphate dehydrogenase deficiency

It has been estimated that there may be as many as a hundred million people in the world who have diminished red cell glucose-6-phosphate dehydrogenase activity. The defective gene is present on the X-chromosome, and thus the clinical features of G6PD deficiency are mainly seen in males ($\overline{X}Y$, where $\overline{X}$ is the abnormal chromosome). Homozygous women ($\overline{X}\overline{X}$) are also clinically affected but such individuals are uncommon. The normal X-chromosome in heterozy-gous women ($\overline{X}X$) usually maintains sufficient G6PD activity to prevent clinical manifestations. The high prevalence of G6PD deficiency must have some Darwinian survival value and there is evidence indicating that deficiency gives some protection to the heterozygous female against *Plasmodium falciparum*;

G6PD deficiency is common only in populations exposed for long periods to tertian malaria and heterozygous females with malaria have lower parasite counts in their red cells than normal women.

Deficiency of the enzyme is found in about 10% of Blacks from West Africa, and is also found to a varying extent in countries around the Mediterranean area, the Middle East, India, Thailand and Southern China. Deficiency is very rare in Caucasians. Of the 300 or so known variants of G6PD, only two are common and these account for over 95% of cases. The most common is the African (or A–) type, where G6PD activities are reduced to about 10% of normal; in the less common Mediterranean type, the enzyme activity is reduced to 1–3%.

Low activities of G6PD result in low concentrations of the reducing compounds NADPH and GSH (see Fig. 3.6). The purpose of these compounds is to maintain haemoglobin and other erythrocytic proteins in a reduced and active form. People with low levels of the enzymes are thus poorly protected against drugs which are oxidants. When oxidants enter the cell they first convert haemoglobin to methaemoglobin and finally denature it so that it precipitates in the red cell in the form of rounded masses known as Heinz bodies (Plate 8). These Heinz bodies (and the portion of the red cell membrane to which they become attached) are removed by splenic macrophages as the red cells pass through the spleen; the resulting inclusion-free cells stain densely, display unstained areas at their periphery ('bite' cells) and undergo extravascular haemolysis. Components of the red-cell membrane may also undergo marked oxidation leading to intravascular haemolysis. Drugs which bring about this type of haemolytic anaemia include the anti-malarial drugs (primaquine), sulphonamides, analgesics such as aspirin (high doses) and phenacetin, and vitamin K analogues.

A number of screening tests and assays for detecting G6PD deficiency are available. These are based on assessing the production of NADPH by red cells in the presence of an excess of glucose-6-phosphate. The NADPH is detected by its ability to reduce Nitro Blue Tetrazolium (NBT) in the presence of an electron transfer agent or to fluoresce in ultraviolet light, or spectrophotometrically.

A variety of clinical syndromes may be associated with G6PD variants which have reduced enzyme activity and these are outlined below.

Episodic acute haemolysis

Most of the time, patients with the two common G6PD variants (A– and Mediterranean types) are symptomless and have normal haemoglobin concentrations. Nevertheless, careful measurement reveals a slight shortening of the red cell life-span. Episodes of haemolytic anaemia develop during infections or following exposure to oxidant drugs and chemicals. Anaemia is maximal about 7–10 days after taking an oxidant. The extent of the fall in haemoglobin concentration is partly dependent on the amount and nature of the drug being given and partly on the extent of reduction of enzyme activity. However, after about 10 days and despite the continuation of the drugs, the haemoglobin concentration rises again and may reach normal levels. This phenomenon is due to the fact that only the older cells, with the lowest G6PD activities, are affected and destroyed by the drug. Heinz bodies may be demonstrated in circulating red cells during the early stages of haemolytic episodes.

Neonatal jaundice

Hyperbilirubinaemia, sometimes necessitating exchange transfusion, has been reported in G6PD-deficient neonates from Greece, Italy, Thailand and China. Such individuals recover completely after the neonatal period but may develop episodic acute haemolysis under the circumstances mentioned above, during later life.

Congenital non-spherocytic haemolytic anaemia

Very rarely, the reduction in G6PD activity is so marked that there is substantial haemolysis and anaemia throughout life.

Favism

Favism has been known for 2000 years or more and is now recognized as an acute haemolytic anaemia occurring in those who have both a deficiency of G6PD (commonly of the Mediterranean type) and also a 'sensitivity' to fava beans. It generally follows ingestion of the broad bean (*Vicia fava*) but may follow inhalation of the pollen, and usually affects children. Severe anaemia develops rapidly and is often accompanied by haemoglobinuria. The biochemical basis of the sensitivity to fava beans has not been identified; favism may affect some G6PD-deficient members of a family but not others.

Abnormalities of the structure or synthesis of haemoglobin

Haemoglobin molecules present in fetal and postnatal life are composed of four polypeptide (globin) chains, two α- and two non-α-chains, which combine together to form a globular protein. Each globin chain is associated with a single haem group which can reversibly combine with oxygen. Most of the haemoglobin in a normal adult is called haemoglobin A (HbA) and consists of two α- and two β-chains ($\alpha_2\beta_2$). Between 1.5 and 3.5% consists of haemoglobin A_2 ($\alpha_2\delta_2$) and less than 1% consists of haemoglobin F or fetal haemoglobin ($\alpha_2\gamma_2$).

Inherited abnormalities of haemoglobin fall into two categories:

1 haemoglobinopathies (structural haemoglobin variants) in which there is an alteration in the amino acid sequence of a globin chain without a reduction in the rate of synthesis of the abnormal chain;

2 thalassaemia syndromes in which there is a depression in the rate of synthesis of one of the globin chains. In the latter, the amino acid sequences of the globin chains are usually normal. However, a thalassaemic blood picture may sometimes arise from the presence of a structurally abnormal globin chain which is synthesized at a reduced rate (e.g. Hb Constant Spring and Hb Lepore) or of an abnormal haemoglobin which is markedly unstable (e.g. Hb Indianapolis).

Structural haemoglobin variants

Over 250 abnormal haemoglobins have been reported but most are rare and only a few lead to clinical or haematological manifestations (Lehmann & Huntsman 1974; Lehmann & Kynoch 1976). The majority of structural haemoglobin variants are the consequence of a single-point mutation affecting one base triplet (codon) in a globin gene and, therefore, have a single amino acid substitution in the affected globin chain (e.g. HbS, HbE, HbC and HbD). If a single-point mutation affects the stop codon of the α-globin gene, the α-chains produced have extra amino acids at one end (e.g. in Hb Constant Spring). A few abnormal haemoglobins result from deletions of one or more base triplets or insertions of extra base triplets and, consequently, show a loss of one or more amino acids or extra amino acids within a chain, respectively. An occasional variant results from fusion genes and contains hybrid chains made of parts of δ- and β-chains (in Hb Lepore) or γ- and β-chains (in Hb Kenya).

The spectrum of clinical and haematological abnormalities that may be caused by abnormal haemoglobins is summarized in Table 3.3. The most common structural haemoglobin variant is haemoglobin S and this is discussed in some detail below. Haemoglobin E is very common in South-East Asia and is found in about 50% of the population in some parts of Thailand. Heterozygotes have about 20–30% HbE, are asymptomatic and are usually not anaemic. They have a low MCV and their blood-films may contain a few target cells. Homozygotes are characterized by mild anaemia, a low MCV and many circulating target cells. Haemoglobin C is confined to people of West African extraction, being present in 7% and 22% of the population in Nigeria and

Different clinical and haematological abnormalities associated with some structural haemoglobin variants.

Variant	Clinical and haematological abnormalities
HbS	Recurrent painful crises (in adults) and chronic haemolytic anaemia; both related to sickling of red cells on deoxygenation*
HbC	Chronic haemolytic anaemia due to reduced red-cell deformability on deoxygenation;* deoxygenated HbC is less soluble than deoxygenated HbA
Hb Köln, Hb Hammersmith	Spontaneous or drug-induced haemolytic anaemia due to instability of the Hb and consequent intracellular precipitation
HbM Boston or HbM Saskatoon	Cyanosis due to congenital methaemoglobinaemia as a consequence of a substitution near or in the haem-pocket
Hb Chesapeake	Hereditary polycythaemia due to increased oxygen affinity
Hb Kansas	Anaemia and cyanosis due to decreased oxygen affinity
Hb Constant Spring, Hb Lepore, HbE	Thalassaemia-like syndrome due to decreased rate of synthesis of abnormal chain
Hb Indianapolis	Thalassaemia-like syndrome due to marked instability of Hb

*Only in homozygotes.

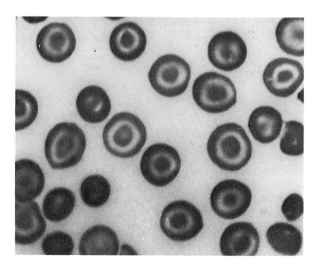

Fig. 3.7 Target cells in the blood film of a homozygote for HbC.

Northern Ghana, respectively. Heterozygotes have 30–40% HbC, are asymptomatic and non-anaemic, and have 6–40% target cells in their blood. Homozygotes have a mild anaemia, low or normal MCV, splenomegaly and many target cells (Fig. 3.7). Haemoglobin S, E and C all result from single amino acid substitutions in the β-chains.

When the amino acid substitution results in an overall change in the charge of the molecule, its migration in a voltage gradient is altered and this can be demonstrated by standard electrophoretic techniques. The speed of migration is characteristic for each abnormal haemoglobin (Fig. 3.8).

Haemoglobin S

In this haemoglobin, the charged glutamic acid residue in position 6 of the normal β-chain is replaced by an uncharged valine molecule. This results in deoxygenated HbS being 50 times less soluble than deoxygenated HbA. The deoxygenated HbS molecules initially polymerise without forming fibres and subsequently polymerize into long fibres (tactoids) (Fig. 3.9) which deform the red cell into the typical sickle-shape (Fig. 3.10). Red cells from heterozygotes for HbS sickle at much lower Po_2 values than those from homozygotes, and do not usually sickle *in vivo*.

The gene for HbS occurs especially in a wide area across tropical Africa, in some countries bordering on the Northern shores of the Mediterranean, and in parts of the Middle East and Southern India (Fig. 3.11). The prevalence of this gene in these areas varies from very low values to 40% of the population. In Black Americans, the prevalence is 8%. The distribution of the HbS gene corresponds to areas in which falciparum malaria has been endemic and the persistence of this potentially lethal gene in high frequency in these areas results from the fact that heterozygotes die less frequently from severe falciparum malaria during early childhood than children with only HbA.

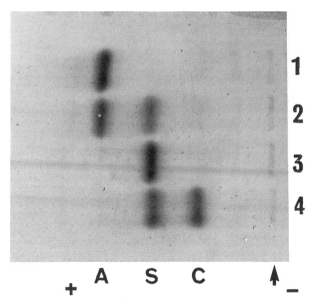

Fig. 3.8 Electrophoresis of haemolysates on cellulose acetate (pH 8.5). (1) Normal adult. (2) Individual with sickle-cell trait; 35% of the haemoglobin consists of HbS and most of the remainder is HbA. (3) Patient with sickle-cell anaemia: most of the haemoglobin is S and there is no A. (4) Double heterozygote for HbS and HbC. This results in a disease which is usually milder than that in homozygotes for HbS.

Sickle-cell trait

Heterozygotes (one gene for HbA and one for HbS) are described as having sickle-cell trait. Their red cells contain between 20 and 45% HbS, the rest beingmainly HbA. They are haematologically normal and are usually asymptomatic. However, spontaneous haematuria may occur occasionally and renal papillary necrosis rarely. Furthermore, there is often an impaired ability to concentrate urine in older individuals. The red cells do not sickle in the trait until the oxygen saturation falls below 40%, a level which is rarely reached in venous blood. Painful crises (see p. 42) and splenic infarction have occurred in severely hypoxic individuals.

Sickle-cell anaemia

Homozygotes for HbS are described as having sickle-cell anaemia. Their red cells contain 80% or more of HbS, the remainder being mainly fetal haemoglobin. The cells sickle at the oxygen tension normally found in venous blood. Initially, there are cycles of sickling and reversal of sickling as the red cells are repeatedly deoxygenated and oxygenated within the circulation. Eventually, irreversibly sickled cells are formed. Both unsickled and sickled red cells containing deoxygenated HbS are less deformable than normal red cells and suffer both extravascular and intravascular haemolysis. The increased rigidity of the cells may cause them to become jammed in and obstruct small and, occasionally, medium-sized blood vessels, thus causing tissue infarction. Symptoms due to infarction are not present continuously but occur in episodes.

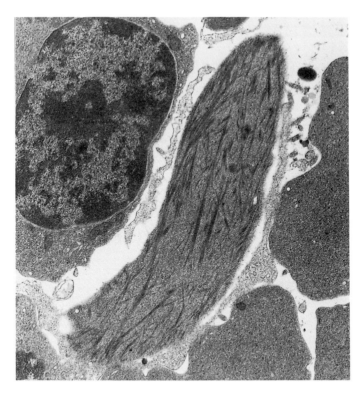

Fig. 3.9 Electron micrograph of a sickled red cell from a homozygote for HbS showing fibres of polymerized deoxygenated HbS running along the long axis of the cell.

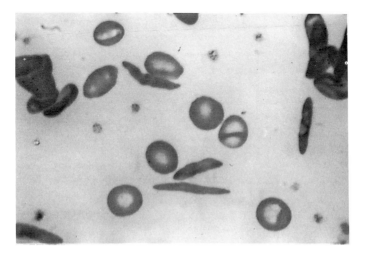

Fig. 3.10 Four sickle cells (with pointed ends) from the blood film of a patient with sickle-cell anaemia (homozygote for HbS).

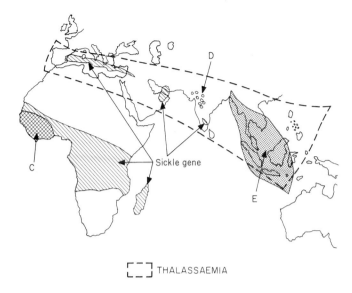

Fig. 3.11   Distribution of the genes for the major haemoglobin variants— S, E, C and D (redrawn from Lehmann & Ager 1960)

There is a chronic haemolytic anaemia at all ages, with the Hb usually varying between 6 and 9 g/dl. Different tissues are particularly liable to infarction at different ages so that the clinical picture varies markedly with age (Sergeant 1976). Furthermore, some patients are only mildly affected having few or no infarctive episodes at any age.

A characteristic feature of sickle-cell anaemia in infancy and early childhood is dactylitis, or the hand–foot syndrome, resulting from occlusion of the nutrient arteries to the metacarpals and metatarsals (Fig. 3.12). There is a painful, non-erythematous and often symmetrical swelling of the hands and feet, lasting 10–14 days. Such infarctive crises may mimic acute rheumatism. Infants and young children may also develop a life-threatening splenic sequestration syndrome. Here there is rapid and extensive trapping of red cells in the spleen leading to profound anaemia, massive splenomegaly, reduced blood volume and hypovolaemic shock. The condition should be treated urgently with blood transfusion.

In older children and adults, recurrent episodes of widespread microvascular occlusion lead to painful crises. These usually consist of attacks of pain affecting the bones and large joints of all four limbs and the back. The crises are accompanied by low-grade fever and may last from a few days to a few weeks. Occasionally the pain may be felt predominantly in one limb or in the chest or abdomen. Patients in this age-group also suffer from larger infarcts affecting the lungs, brain and bones (leading to avascular necrosis of the heads of the femora or humeri and of the diaphyses of long bones). Other clinical features include chronic leg ulcers (Fig. 3.13) and priapism. The spleen is usually palpable in children, but it atrophies from repeated infarction and is usually not felt in adults. Almost all the patients show abnormalities of retinal vessels on ophthalmoscopy.

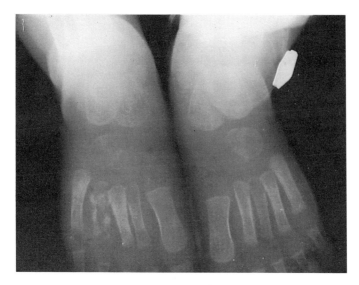

Fig. 3.12 X-ray of the feet of a child with sickle-cell anaemia 2 weeks after the onset of the hand–foot syndrome, showing necrosis of the right fourth metatarsal.

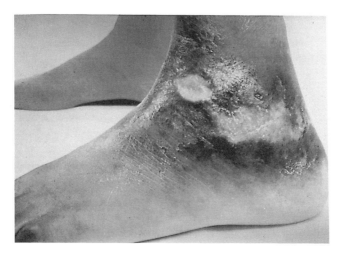

Fig. 3.13 Chronic leg ulcer with increased pigmentation of the surrounding skin in a woman with sickle-cell anaemia.

Aplastic crises due to parvovirus infection may occur (p. 29) as may an aggravation of the anaemia due to a secondary folate deficiency (p. 98).

There is an increased susceptibility to fulminant bacterial infections apparently due to a combination of hyposplenism and an abnormality in opsonization.

There is a high early mortality rate, the magnitude of which is dependent on the quality of health care and on living conditions. In a prospective survey in Jamaica (Rogers *et al.* 1978) 13% of the children died in the first 2 years of life. The principal causes of death were acute splenic sequestration of red cells and pneumococcal sepsis (meningitis, pneumonia, septicaemia), both of extremely rapid onset, but both amenable to treatment.

Many patients with sickle-cell anaemia have at least a few sickled cells in their blood film but others do not. The diagnosis is made by finding (a) a positive result with a screening test for HbS (e.g. sickling or solubility test); (b) a single major band moving in the position of HbS on electrophoresis both at an alkaline and acid pH (see Fig. 3.8); and (c) the sickle-cell trait in both parents. Heterozygotes for HbS also give a positive result with screening tests for HbS but do not have sickled cells on their blood films, and show a mixture of HbA and S on electrophoresis.

Thalassaemia

A comprehensive account of the thalassaemia syndromes is found in the monograph by Weatherall and Clegg (1981). The thalassaemias are broadly divided into two main groups, the α-thalassaemias and the β-thalassaemias, depending on whether the defect lies in the synthesis of α- or β-globin chains, respectively.

Alpha-thalassaemias

The α-thalassaemias are seen with greatest frequency in Southeast Asia (Thailand, Malay peninsula and Indonesia), the Mediterranean region, the Middle East, and West Africa. Sporadic cases have been reported in most racial groups. There are two closely linked α-globin genes on chromosome 16 and thus four α-globin genes per cell. In most Asian patients with the α-thalassaemia syndromes, the primary biochemical defect is a deletion of one, two, three or all four of the α-globin genes. However, dysfunctional rather than completely deleted genes may also be found; these are caused by partial deletions or non-deletional defects (usually a single-base change) and are particularly seen in Thailand and Saudi Arabia. The manifestations of α-thalassaemia depend on the number of genes deleted in a particular individual. Deletion of one or two genes causes an asymptomatic condition with minor haematological changes and deletion of three and four genes causes HbH disease and Hb Bart's hydrops fetalis syndrome, respectively. There are two main varieties of abnormal chromosome (Fig. 3.14). In the first, one of the two genes on a chromosome may be deleted (α^+-thalassaemia determinant) and in the second, both genes may be deleted (α^0-thalassaemia determinant). Both the α^0-thalassaemia and the α^+-thalassaemia determinants are found in Southeast Asia and the Mediterranean region. The main type of α-thalassaemia determinant found in West Africa, India and the Pacific Islands is α^+; α^0 is very rare. In populations in which the α^0-thalassaemia determinant is rare, haemoglobin H disease is rare and Hb Bart's hydrops fetalis syndrome is not found. In Northern Thailand, where both the α^+ and α^0 determinants are particularly common, 0.4% of deliveries are stillbirths due to Hb Bart's hydrops fetalis syndrome and HbH disease is found in about 1% of the population.

α^+ thalassaemia trait (deletion of one gene)

This condition is seen when the α^+-thalassaemia determinant is present on

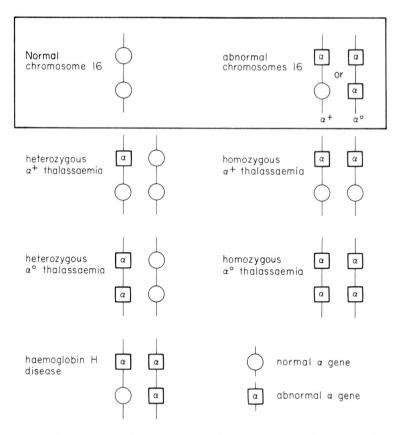

Fig. 3.14 Diagram to show how the two forms of abnormal chromosome 16 (α^+ and α^0) are arranged to give the different forms of α-thalassaemia. Homozygotes for α^0-thalassaemia suffer from Hb Bart's hydrops fetalis syndrome.

only one of the number 16 chromosomes (i.e. in heterozygotes for the α^+ determinant). Patients are asymptomatic but may be slightly anaemic. About 15% show slight reductions in MCV and MCH.

α^0 *thalassaemia trait (deletion of two genes)*

This is seen in two circumstances, either in homozygotes for the α^+-thalassaemia determinant or in heterozygotes for the α^0-thalassaemia determinant. Similar haematological changes are seen in both situations. The Hb is either normal or slightly reduced and the MCV and MCH are usually reduced.

Haemoglobin H disease (deletion of three genes)

This chronic haemolytic anaemia results from the presence of both the α^+- and α^0-thalassaemia determinants. α-chains are produced at very low rates and there is a considerable excess of β-chains which combine to form tetramers (β_4). This tretramer is known as haemoglobin H. Haemoglobin H is unstable and precipitates as the erythrocytes get older, forming rigid Heinz bodies (Plate 8) which are removed during passage of affected red cells through the spleen. The damage to the membrane brought about by this removal results in a shortened red cell life-span. The clinical picture of haemoglobin H disease is very variable. Most patients are moderately affected with a condition similar to β-thalassaemia intermedia while some are more severely affected and others are only mildly affected and live almost normal lives. Splenomegaly is seen in most patients. The Hb concentration is usually between 7 and 11 g/dl but may be as low as 3–4 g/dl; the red cells are hypochromic and show variation in size and shape. Both the MCV and MCH are reduced.

Hb Bart's hydrops fetalis syndrome (deletion of four genes)

This occurs when there is homozygosity for the α^0-thalassaemia determinant. No α-chains can be formed and the predominant chain synthesized is the γ-chain, which forms tetramers (γ_4, haemoglobin Bart's). There is persistence in the fetus of the embryonic haemoglobin, Hb Portland ($\zeta_2\gamma_2$). Intrauterine death followed by a stillbirth usually occurs between 25 and 40 weeks of gestation, or the baby dies very shortly after birth.

Beta-thalassaemias

Beta-thalassaemia has a worldwide distribution. It is frequently seen in the Mediterranean region and in parts of the Middle-East, India, Pakistan and South-East Asia; in these areas, the carrier frequencies vary between 2 and 30%. It has been suggested that the high prevalence of the β-thalassaemia gene in these regions results from the gene bestowing a protective effect against *P. falciparum* on heterozygotes.

The β-thalassaemias result from a large number of different genetic abnormalities (Kazazian *et al.* 1986); the prevalence of particular abnormalities varies between different races. The β-chain genes are usually not completely deleted but often show single nucleotide substitutions or additions or small deletions. In some cases, no mRNA is produced from the abnormal gene at all, in others there is a reduced production, and in some, structurally and/or functionally abnormal mRNA is transcribed but not translated into whole β-chains. Patients in whom the genetic abnormality causes an absence of β-chain production are described as having β^0-thalassaemia and those in whom the abnormality causes a reduction in the rate of β-chain production are described as having β^+-thalassaemia. The β^0 type predominates in India and Pakistan, the β^+ type predominates in Sardinia and Cyprus and both types are found in Greece, the Middle-East and Thailand.

Heterozygous β-thalassaemia

Most affected subjects are asymptomatic. The haemoglobin concentration is either normal (thalassaemia minima) or slightly reduced (thalassaemia minor), the red cell count is high and the MCV is usually low. The Romanowsky-stained blood-film shows microcytosis, target cells and red cells with basophilic stippling (i.e. several fine or coarse bluish-black granules consisting of aggregated ribosomes). The HbA$_2$ level is raised to 3.5–7.0% and half the cases show slightly increased HbF levels, which are in the range 1–5%. Serum iron, total iron-binding capacity and serum ferritin are normal in the absence of co-existing iron deficiency.

Homozygous β-thalassaemia

This condition causes one of two syndromes, one characterized by severe anaemia usually developing between the second and twelfth months of life (β-thalassaemia major) and the other by moderate anaemia developing after the age of 1–2 years (β-thalassaemia intermedia). The inability to produce β-chains leads to the presence of an excess of α-chains in early and late polychromatic erythroblasts. The α-chains precipitate within the cells and this leads to an impairment of various cellular functions and the phagocytosis and degradation of a proportion of the precipitate-containing erythroblasts by bone marrow macrophages (ineffective erythropoiesis) (Wickramasinghe 1976). There is also a considerably shortened survival of precipitate-containing red cells which enter the circulation so that the anaemia results from a combination of ineffective erythropoiesis and peripheral haemolysis. The response to the anaemia and ineffective erythropoiesis is an enormous erythroid hyperplasia which results in skeletal changes mainly affecting the skull, long bones and hands.

β-thalassaemia major (Cooley's anaemia)

This disease does not present at birth since production of fetal haemoglobin, $\alpha_2\gamma_2$, is not affected. The infant becomes profoundly anaemic (Hb concentration 2.5–6.5 g/dl) and mildly jaundiced after the first few months of life, at the time when HbA should be replacing HbF. There is also failure to thrive, abdominal enlargement due to hepatosplenomegaly, and recurrent fever. If a transfusion programme is not instituted, growth is retarded, the abdomen becomes more enlarged, muscle development is poor and various skeletal deformities due to the gross expansion of erythropoietic tissue appear. The skeletal changes cause the typical 'thalassaemic' facies with frontal and parietal bossing, enlargement of the maxillary bones causing severe dental deformities and malocclusion of the teeth, and depression of the bridge of the nose. The long bones and bones of the hands show thinning of the cortex. Fractures of long bones are frequent and may be the presenting sign. X-ray of the skull shows enlargement of the diploic spaces and radiating striations in the subperiosteal bone ('hair-on-end' appearance).

The excessive red-cell destruction (due to deposits of α-chain in the red cells) causes considerable enlargement of the spleen, and this itself may aggravate the anaemia due to increased pooling of red cells in that organ, an expanded plasma volume and secondary hypersplenism with a further shortening of red cell life-span. The hypersplenism also causes neutropenia and thrombocytopenia.

Iron absorption from the gut is excessive, and this, together with the regular blood transfusions (each unit of blood contains 200 mg iron) causes haemosiderosis, from which the patients usually die between the ages of 10 and 20 years. Iron deposition causes cirrhosis of the liver, diabetes mellitus and myocardial damage leading to fatal arrhythmias or congestive cardiac failure. The iron deposition also causes endocrine dysfunction and leads to a failure to grow normally during puberty and a failure to develop secondary sexual characteristics.

The peripheral blood contains microcytic hypochromic red cells which also vary greatly in size and shape, and target cells (Fig. 3.15). The serum iron

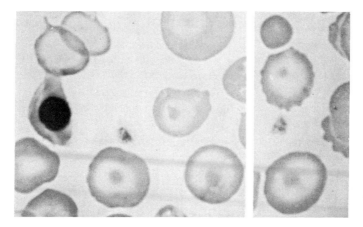

Fig. 3.15 Target cells, hypochromic red cells and an erythroblast from the peripheral blood film of a patient with homozygous β-thalassaemia.

concentration is high, the total iron-binding capacity is usually low and the iron-binding protein, transferrin, almost completely saturated with iron. Electrophoresis of haemoglobin shows that more than 50% is HbF. There is an absence or reduction of HbA, depending on whether the abnormal genes are of the β^0 or β^+ type.

Treatment of β-thalassaemia major

It is not possible appreciably to alter globin chain production at the present time and therapy centres around regular transfusion about every 4–6 weeks, such that the Hb concentration is always maintained above 11 g/dl. With this treatment, children grow and mature normally and lead normal lives (Modell 1976). If the spleen is considerably enlarged and there is clear evidence that it is also trapping the transfused red cells and increasing transfusion requirements, then splenectomy is carried out. An important aspect of modern treatment is the reduction of tissue damage due to haemosiderosis by the daily administration of the iron-chelating agent, desferrioxamine. This agent is given subcutaneously overnight using a portable pump and has been shown to limit iron accumulation and prolong life.

Antenatal diagnosis of β-thalassaemia

It is possible to make an antenatal diagnosis of homozygous β-thalassaemia on blood obtained from a 18–20-week-old fetus. The reticulocytes are analysed for β-chain production and the diagnosis of homozygous β-thalassaemia is made when β-chain production is absent or markedly reduced. Parents often decide to abort homozygous fetuses. Antenatal diagnosis can be made much earlier during pregnancy (i.e. at 9–11 weeks) from an analysis of chorionic villous or amniocyte DNA either directly by using oligonucleotide probes complementary to specific mutations or indirectly by linkage analysis with polymorphic restriction sites at the β-globin gene cluster.

β-thalassaemia intermedia

Most patients with this condition are reasonably well and require transfusions only during intercurrent infections. Clinical features include skeletal deformities (see p. 46), splenomegaly (which may become sufficiently marked to require splenectomy), formation of masses of extramedullary haemopoietic tissue which may cause pressure symptoms, recurrent leg ulcers, and haemosiderosis in adult life due to increased iron absorption. The clinical picture of thalassaemia intermedia arises not only from homozygosity for the β^+ thalassaemia gene but also from interactions between β-thalassaemia and other genetic abnormalities (e.g. α-thalassemia, δβ-thalassaemia and Hb Lepore).

ACQUIRED HAEMOLYTIC ANAEMIAS

Red cells may be destroyed either by immunological or by non-immunological mechanisms.

Immune haemolytic anaemias

In these conditions, red cells react with antibody with or without complement activation and are consequently destroyed. IgG-coated red cells interact with the Fc receptors on macrophages and are then either completely or partially phagocytosed. When the phagocytosis is partial, the unphagocytosed part of the cell may detach from the macrophage and circulate as a spherocyte. Red cells which are also coated with the activated complement component C3 interact with C3 receptors on macrophages and are, usually, completely phagocytosed. In most instances where complement is activated, the cascade sequence only proceeds as far as C3 deposition on the cell surface. In a few instances, activation of complement is more intense and proceeds as far as deposition of the membrane attack complex (C5–C9) which results in intravascular haemolysis. The immune haemolytic anaemias include haemolytic transfusion reactions (p. 193), haemolytic disease of the newborn (p. 55), autoimmune haemolytic anaemias and some drug-related haemolytic anaemias. In paroxysmal nocturnal haemoglobinuria, there is an acquired defect in the red cell membrane which leads to complement-mediated haemolysis.

Autoimmune haemolytic anaemias

A classification of the autoimmune haemolytic anaemias is given in Table 3.4.

The antibody found in these patients can be subdivided into two character-istic types, 'warm' antibody and 'cold' antibody (Dacie 1959). A 'warm' antibody reacts best with the red cell at 37°C and does not bring about agglutination. A 'cold' antibody reacts best only at a temperture below 32°C and usually agglutinates the red cells. The clinical picture associated with the two types is different.

Autoimmune haemolytic anaemia (AIHA) with warm-reactive antibodies

Patients are usually over the age of 50 years. In the idiopathic condition haemolysis dominates the clinical picture, and no evidence can be found of any other disease. In the secondary condition, the haemolysis is associated with a

Table 3.4   Classification of autoimmune haemolytic anaemias.

Caused by warm-reactive antibodies
Idiopathic
Secondary (chronic lymphocytic leukaemia, lymphoma, other
   malignant tumours, SLE)

Caused by cold-reactive antibodies
Cold haemagglutinin disease
   Idiopathic
   Secondary (*Mycoplasma pneumoniae*
      infection, infectious mononucleosis, lymphomas)

Paroxysmal cold haemoglobinuria
   Idiopathic
   Secondary (some viral infections, congenital and tertiary
      syphilis)

---

primary disease such as chronic lymphocytic leukaemia and systemic lupus erythematosus. In most patients the nature of the antigen on the red cell with which the autoantibody reacts cannot be determined, but in a few patients the antibody reacts with some of the antigens of the Rh system.

Symptoms are unrelated to ambient temperature. The clinical presentation is extremely variable. Some patients are very ill with an acute onset of severe anaemia and others have few or no symptoms and a mild chronic anaemia or even a compensated haemolytic state. Mild jaundice is common and spleno-megaly is almost always found.

Haematological findings include anaemia, spherocytosis (Fig. 3.16), reticu-locytosis, erythroblastaemia and neutrophil leucocytosis. IgG, complement

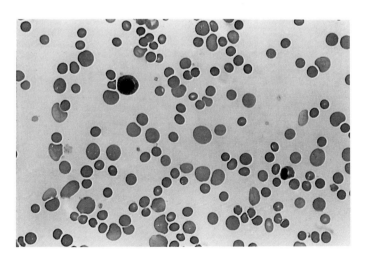

Fig. 3.16   Blood film from a patient with idiopathic autoimmune haemolytic anaemia (warm-reactive antibody). In addition to several microspherocytes, the photomicrograph shows two erythroblasts.

components or both can usually be detected on the red cells using a direct antiglobulin test.

In most patients, the haemolysis can be reduced by treatment with prednisolone, which is initially given in high doses. If there is no response to steroids or if the reduction in haemolysis is not maintained when the dose of steroids is decreased, splenectomy or immunosuppressive therapy with drugs such as azathioprine or cyclophosphamide should be tried and may be beneficial.

Cold haemagglutinin disease (CHAD)

Since cold antibody only reacts with red cells at a temperature below about 32°C, symptoms are worse during cold weather; skin temperature frequently falls well below 32°C when exposed to the cold. Exposure to cold provokes acrocyanosis (coldness, purplish discolouration and numbness of fingers, toes, ear lobes and the nose). This symptom is due to the formation of agglutinates of red cells in the vessels of the skin. Cold antibody attached to red cells also activates the complement system and leads to red cell lysis and, consequently, to haemoglobinaemia and haemoglobinuria.

Blood films made at room temperature show large red-cell agglutinates (Fig. 3.17). The cold agglutinin in chronic idiopathic CHAD is usually a monoclonal IgM antibody usually with anti-I specificity. The anti-I titre at 4°C may be as high as 1:2 000–1:500 000 (normal, 1:10–40).

Rarely, patients with *Mycoplasma* pneumonia or infectious mononucleosis may develop acute self-limiting cold haemagglutinin disease due to the production of polyclonal IgM antibodies with anti-I or anti-i specificity, respectively.

Chronic idiopathic CHAD is treated by keeping the patient warm during the winter and, if necessary, by the use of chlorambucil or cyclophosphamide.

Paroxysmal cold haemoglobinuria

This rare disease is caused by an IgG antibody with anti-P specificity. This antibody is capable of binding complement and is called the Donath–Landsteiner

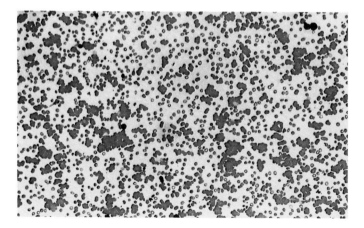

Fig. 3.17 Numerous red-cell agglutinates on a blood film from a patient with idiopathic cold haemagglutinin disease.

antibody. Patients suffer from acute episodes of marked haemoglobinuria due to severe intravascular haemolysis when exposed to the cold. The diagnosis is based on serological studies demonstrating the presence of this particular antibody. A rapid screening test consists of incubating the patient's red cells and serum at $0-4°C$ and then warming the mixture to $37°C$. Antibody and early complement components bind to red cells at $0-4°C$ but lysis occurs only on warming to $37°C$ (Donath–Landsteiner test).

Paroxysmal nocturnal haemoglobinuria (PNH)

This is an acquired disease in which an abnormal clone of haemopoietic cells derived from a multipotent stem cell gives rise to erythrocytes, leucocytes and platelets with a defect in the cell membrane. The defect involves a membrane protein concerned with complement inactivation and, therefore, protection of the cells against inadvertent lysis. The affected cells are thus unusually sensitive to lysis by the terminal complement complex (C5–C9). The essential features of the disease are intravascular haemolysis, recurrent venous thrombosis and pancytopenia. The haemolysis is usually mild and chronic but may be severe and episodic with haemoglobulinuria, which is predominantly nocturnal. The PNH defect may occasionally develop during the course of aplastic anaemia. It may also precede marrow aplasia or develop after recovery from aplasia. Some cases of PNH terminate in leukaemia. The diagnosis is usually based on the susceptibility of PNH red cells to undergo lysis when incubated with acidified fresh autologous serum (acidified serum lysis test or Ham test).

Non-immune haemolytic anaemias

A comprehensive account of this group of haemolytic anaemias is given by Wintrobe *et al.* (1981). Several causes of non-immune haemolytic anaemia are summarized in Table 3.5. Some drugs cause haemolysis by non-immune mechanisms and others by immune mechanisms; haemolytic anaemias due to drugs are considered in the following section.

Haemolytic anaemia due to drugs

Any drug which affects essential structural components or functional activities of a red cell is likely to cause a shortening of red cell life-span. It is not surprising, therefore, that a large number of drugs have been reported to cause haemolysis. When any haemolytic anaemia is encountered, it is necessary to enquire closely to determine whether there has been any exposure to drugs or chemicals (Dacie 1962; Worlledge *et al.* 1982).

The precise way in which many drugs act on the red cell is not known, but five categories of action can be recognized:

1   Certain chemicals, such as benzene, toluene and saponin, which are fat-solvents, act on the red cell membrane and disrupt its lipid components.

2   Certain drugs, such as primaquine, sulphonamides and phenacetin oxidize and denature haemoglobin and other cell components in people with a deficiency of G6PD or some other red-cell enzymes (p. 34). However, if given in a large enough dose these drugs also affect normal red cells. When given in

Table 3.5 Causes of non-immune haemolytic anaemias.

Mechanical trauma to red cells
Red cell fragmentation due to abnormalities in the heart and large
    blood vessels (aortic valve prostheses, severe aortic valve
    disease, extensive dissecting aneurysms of the aorta)

Microangiopathic haemolytic anaemia (haemolytic uraemic syndrome,
    thrombotic thrombocytopenic purpura, metastatic malignancy,
    malignant hypertension, disseminated intravascular
    coagulation, giant haemangioma)

March haemoglobinuria

Burns

Infections
Septicaemias due to *Clostridium perfringens* (*welchii*) or various
    cocci, leptospirosis, malaria (Fig. 3.18), toxoplasmosis,
    bartonellosis

Drugs,* chemicals and venoms*
Oxidant drugs and chemicals, arsine, venoms of certain spiders and
    snakes

Hypersplenism

*Some drugs cause haemolysis by immune mechanisms.

conventional doses, the two oxidant drugs dapsone and sulphasalazine cause haemolysis in most patients.

3   There are drugs which combine with components on the surface of the red cell and generate complexes which act as antigens. The resulting antibody then reacts with the drug-cell surface complex and brings about red-cell destruction. Penicillin, when given in very large doses (more than 6 g/day), can occasionally cause a haemolytic anaemia in this way (White *et al* 1968).

4   Certain drugs, such as stibophen, become antigenic after combining with serum proteins. The antibodies that are produced form circulating antigen–antibody complexes which become adsorbed onto the red cell surface. The adsorbed antigen–antibody complexes activate complement and cause lysis of the affected red cells (the 'innocent-bystander' mechanism).

5   Finally, methyldopa and mefenamic or flufenamic acid trigger the development of an autoimmune haemolytic anaemia associated with warm-reactive autoantibodies, perhaps by an effect of the drug on suppressor T-lymphocytes.

OBJECTIVES IN LEARNING

1   To know the tests for recognizing:
    (a) that red cells are being destroyed at an excessive rate;
    (b) that the marrow is producing cells at a rate in excess of normal.

2   To know the division of haemolytic anaemias into congenital and acquired and to know the aetiological factors in each division.

3   To understand the following aspects of hereditary spherocytosis:

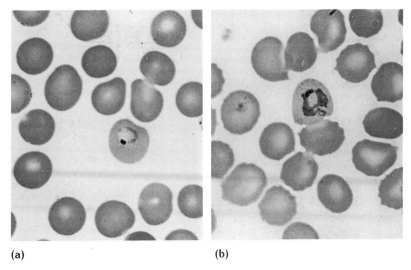

(a) (b)

Fig. 3.18 Peripheral blood-film from a patient with *Plasmodium vivax* malaria showing two parasitized red cells each containing a single parasite. (a) Ring form (early trophozoite) within a slightly enlarged red cell. (b) Amoeboid late trophozoite; the parasitized cell is enlarged and stippled. The ring forms of *Plasmodium falciparum* are smaller and more delicate than those of *Plasmodium vivax* and do not cause enlargement of the parasitized red cells. Especially in falciparum malaria, more than one parasite may be found within a single red cell.

    (a) mode of inheritance;
    (b) clinical features and modes of presentation;
    (c) laboratory findings specific for this disease.

4 To understand the role of glucose-6-phosphate dehydrogenase in glucose metabolism and the pathogenesis and clinical characteristics of the haemolytic syndromes which may be associated with a deficiency of this enzyme.

5 To understand the ways in which abnormalities in the structure and rate of synthesis of globin chains cause clinical and haematological abnormalities and to know the clinical and laboratory manifestations of sickle-cell anaemia and the common thalassaemia syndromes.

6 To understand the role of autoantibodies in the production of haemolytic anaemias and to know the types of disease with which they are associated.

7 To know some of the causes of non-immune acquired haemolytic anaemias.

REFERENCES

Agre P., Asimos A., Casella J.F., McMillan, C. (1986) Inheritance pattern and clinical response to splenectomy as a reflection of erythrocyte spectrin deficiency in hereditary spherocytosis. *N. Eng. J. Med.*, **315**: 1579.

Beutler E. (1959) The hemolytic effect of primaquine and related compounds: a review. *Blood*, **14**: 103.

Dacie J.V. (1959) Acquired haemolytic anaemias. *Br. Med. Bull.*, **15**; 67.

Dacie J.V. (1962) Haemolytic reactions to drugs. *Proc. R. Soc. Med.*, **55**: 28.

Dacie J.V. (1967) *The Haemolytic Anaemias* (2nd edn). Parts III and IV. Churchill, London.

Dacie J.V. (1985) *The Haemolytic Anaemias*, 3rd edn, Vol 1: *The Hereditary Anaemias*, Part I. Churchill Livingstone, Edinburgh.
Dacie J. (1988) *The Haemolytic Anaemias*, 3rd edn, Vol 2; *The Hereditary Anaemias*, Part 2. Churchill Livingstone, Edinburgh.
Haden R.L. (1947) A new type of hereditary haemolytic jaundice without spherocytosis. *Am. J. Med. Sci.*, **214**: 255.
Kazazian H.H., Jr., Dowling C.E., Waber P.G., Huang S., Lo W.H.Y. (1986) The spectrum of β-thalassaemia genes in China and Southeast Asia. *Blood* **68**: 964.
Lehmann H., Ager J.A.M. (1960) In: *The Metabolic Basis of Inherited Disease*. (eds. Stanbury *et al.*) McGraw Hill, New York.
Lehmann H., Huntsman R.G. (1974) *Man's Haemoglobins*. North Holland Publishing Company, Amsterdam.
Lehmann H., Kynoch P.A.M. (1976) *Human Haemoglobin Variants and their Characteristics*. North Holland Publishing Company, Amsterdam.
Mackinney A.A. (1965) Hereditary spherocytosis. *Arch. Intern. Med.*, **116**: 257.
Mentzer W.C. (ed.) (1981) Enzymopathies. *Clinics in Haematology*, Vol 10.1. W.B. Saunders, Philadelphia.
Modell B. (1976) Management of thalassaemia major. *Br. Med. Bull.*, **32**: 270.
Mollison P.L. Engelfriet C.P., Contreras M. (1987) *Blood Transfusion in Clinical Medicine* (8th edn). Blackwell Scientific Publications, Oxford.
Palek J. (1985) Hereditary elliptocytosis and related disorders. *Clin. Haematol.* **14**: 45.
Rogers D.W., Clarke J.M., Cupidore L., Ramlal A.M., Sparke B.R., Serjeant G.R. (1978) Early deaths in Jamaican children with sickle-cell disease. *Br. Med. J.*, **1**: 1515.
Sergeant G. (1976) *Sickle-Cell Anaemia*. North Holland Publications, Amsterdam.
Weatherall D.J., Clegg J.B. (1981) *The Thalassaemia Syndromes* (3rd edn). Blackwell Scientific Publications, Oxford.
White J.M., Brown D.L., Hepner G.W., Worlledge S.M. (1968) Penicillin-induced haemolytic anaemia. *Br. Med. J.*, **3**: 26.
Wickramasinghe S.N. (1976) The morphology and kinetics of erythropoiesis in homozygous β-thalassaemia, Ciba Foundation Symposium 37 (new Proceedings of series) on *Congenital Disorders of Erythropoiesis* (eds R. Porter and D.W. Fitzsimons), pp. 221–243. Elsevier, Amsterdam.
Wintrobe M.M. Lee G.R., Boggs D.R., Bithell T.C., Foerster J., Athens J. W., Lukens J.N. (1981) *Clinical Hematology* (8th edn). Lea & Febiger, Philadelphia.
Worlledge S., Hughes-Jones N.C., Bain B. (1982) Immune haemolytic anaemias. In: *Blood and its Disorder* (eds R.M. Hardisty & D.J. Weatherall), p. 479. Blackwell Scientific Publications, Oxford.

RECOMMENDED READING

Allgood J.W., Chaplin H. (1967) Idiopathic acquired autoimmune hemolytic anemia. A review of forty-seven cases treated from 1955 through 1965. *Am. J. Med.*, **43**: 254.
Editorial (1969) Glucose-6-phosphate dehydrogenase deficiency and favism. *Lancet*, ii, 1177.

Chapter 4
Haemolytic Disease of the Newborn

Haemolytic disease of the newborn (HDN) is the result of the transplacental passage of maternal blood-group antibodies, which become attached to the fetal cells and cause their destruction. In almost all clinically affected cases, the antibody concerned is within the Rh blood-group system. Giblett (1964) found that 93% of such cases were due to anti-D, 6% to anti-c or anti-E, and only the remaining 1% were due to antibodies of other blood-group systems, including the ABO system. Without treatment, the mortality rate of affected infants is about 20%, but the antenatal prediction of the disease, together with the introduction of treatment by exchange transfusion has considerably reduced this value. Approximately 60% of affected infants require an exchange transfusion and in the best hands efficient treatment results in the survival of about 95% of all those who are born alive. Nevertheless, during the decade 1958–68, the disease resulted in about 300–400 neonatal deaths each year in Britain and approximately an equal number were stillborn. The introduction during 1968 of prophylactic injections of anti-D into the mother immediately after labour to prevent active immunization has greatly reduced the incidence of haemolytic disease of the newborn. In the mid 1980s, only about 20–40 deaths occurred each year in the UK. Nevertheless, it is most important that antenatal prediction of the occurrence of the disease should continue to be made, since it is unlikely that complete suppression of immunization can be brought about. A low mortality rate can only be maintained if those who are born with the disease are treated within a few hours of birth. Once an Rh-negative mother (genotype *cde/cde*) has anti-D in her plasma there is no known way of inhibiting this production and all subsequent Rh-positive infants (those with the *D* gene) will be affected.

HAEMOLYTIC DISEASE DUE TO ANTI-D

The aetiology of haemolytic disease of the newborn was first elucidated by Levine *et al.* (1941). A mother who had given birth to an affected infant was transfused with her husband's blood and this was followed by a transfusion reaction. The authors correctly surmised that the mother had been immunized by a fetal antigen which had been derived from the father.

The Rh-antigens are only present on red cells and it is the passage of red cells from the fetus across the placenta into the mother that gives rise to the immunization of the mother in the first place. Direct evidence for the presence of fetal red cells in the maternal circulation has been obtained using the acid-elution (Kleihauer) technique in which a dried film of maternal blood on a glass slide is dipped into a buffer solution at pH 3.5. Adult haemoglobin is soluble in this solution but fetal haemoglobin is not, so that subsequent counter-staining demonstrates the intact fetal red cells amongst a background of pale haemoglobin-free maternal cells (Fig. 4.1). Fetal cells can occasionally be found in the maternal circulation during pregnancy, especially during the third trimester, but transplacental passage occurs mainly at the time of labour. About 15% of women have been shown to have more than 0.1 ml of fetal red cells in the circulation after labour and occasionally the number of cells may exceed 50 ml. There is evidence that the greater the number of fetal cells in the circulation after labour, the greater the chance of developing antibodies (Clarke 1967, 1968). Relationship between the total amount of fetal red cells in the maternal circulation immediately after labour and the incidence of immunization of mothers 6 months later is shown in Table 4.1.

In a Caucasian population, about 17% of the women are Rh-negative. The fathers of the children born to these mothers will be either homozygous for *D* (*DD*), heterozygous for *D* (*Dd*), or *dd*, and it can be calculated that only about 50% of all mothers who are Rh-negative will give birth to 2 successive Rh-positive infants. In theory then, the incidence of HDN should be 8% of all second pregnancies, but in practice the incidence was only about 1% before the advent of preventive therapy. This results from the fact that frequently the amount of fetal red cells crossing the placenta is insufficient to initiate immunization, combined with the fact that only some 60–70% of Rh-negative mothers are able to respond to the D-antigen by producing anti-D.

It is very unusual for the first-born child to be affected with HDN, the incidence being slightly less than 1% of all Rh-negative mothers with no history of transfusion or abortion. The reason for this is that it is only occasionally that significant numbers of fetal red cells cross the placenta sufficiently early in pregnancy to stimulate anti-D production before the child is born. The total incidence of HDN in first born children is nevertheless higher than 1%, as a number of mothers become immunized through abortion or miscarriage or by transfusion of Rh-positive blood.

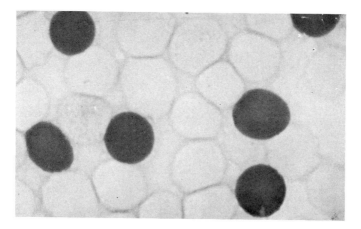

Fig. 4.1 Post-partum maternal blood film, stained by the acid elution technique of Kleihauer. The darkly-staining cells are fetal red cells present in the maternal circulation. The mother's cells have lost their haemoglobin and appear very pale.

Table 4.1 Relationship between fetal red cells in the maternal circulation after labour and subsequent immunization of mother (adapted from Clarke 1968).

Estimated number of fetalred cells (ml)	Incidence of immunization (%)
0	3.7
0.02	4.5
0.04	10.3
0.06–0.08	14.6
0.1–0.2	18.7
0.22–0.78	21.1
>0.8	23.5

If the fetal red cells in the mother after labour bring about a primary immunization, antibody may be detected within the following 6 months. In about half the cases, however, antibody concentrations do not rise sufficiently high for anti-D to be detected at this time by the antiglobulin test. During the subsequent pregnancy with an Rh-positive fetus, a few fetal red cells crossing the placenta early in pregnancy provide a secondary stimulus to anti-D production, which can usually be detected by the 28th week but may not appear until the last few weeks of pregnancy.

Anti-D may belong to either the IgM or IgG immunoglobulin class. It is only the IgG class that is actively transferred across the placenta to the fetus. IgM anti-D is relatively rare, and does not cross the placenta.

Mothers who lack the c or E antigens, for example, those whose genotype is *CDe/CDe*, can produce anti-c or anti-E if red cells containing the C or E antigens cross the placenta. The incidence of these antibodies is low and if they are to be detected antenatally, it is necessary to look for them in both Rh-positive and negative mothers. Since this involves a great deal of laboratory work, it is only carried out at a few centres.

Clinical features

There is a very great variation in the severity of the disease in the child. At one end of the scale there are infants who are not anaemic at all at birth and who never become jaundiced. However, the haemoglobin concentration of these infants may fall abnormally rapidly after birth and values as low as 6 g/dl may be found up to 30 days later. All neonates with antibodies on their red cells (positive antiglobulin test) should therefore be followed up for 1 month after birth.

The overall severity of the disease in a family with several affected infants usually tends to be consistent, the infants are either all mildly or all severely affected. Moderately severely affected babies may or may not be anaemic at birth, but the rate of red-cell destruction is such that jaundice develops within a few hours. Jaundice is not seen at the time of birth since prior to this the bilirubin is excreted by placental transfer. Within 48–72 hours of birth, the plasma bilirubin may rise to 350–700 μmol/l. The rate of rise of plasma bilirubin is governed partly by the rate of red-cell destruction and partly by the degree of maturity of the bilirubin excretory mechanism, that is, on the state of development of glucuronyl transferase. As a result of the poor development of the excretory mechanism for bilirubin in many infants, it is quite common for a child with a cord haemoglobin within the normal range (lower limit 13.5 g/dl) to become severely jaundiced. The danger associated with a high bilirubin level is kernicterus (i.e. staining of and damage to the basal ganglia of the brain), with a clinical picture characterized by spasticity, arched back and death from respiratory failure. Those that survive usually have a subnormal intelligence.

Severely affected babies become so anaemic that they develop cardiac failure and are either stillborn or die shortly after birth, although those with mild cardiac failure can be resuscitated by exchange transfusion. Apart from anaemia, the characteristic feature of these children is oedema. The stillbirth rate is approximately 15% of all fetuses with haemolytic disease and death may occur from the 20th week onwards.

HAEMOLYTIC DISEASE DUE TO ANTI-A AND ANTI-B

Haemolytic disease due to anti-A or anti-B is almost entirely confined to group A and B infants born to group O mothers, since it is mainly group O mothers who have anti-A and anti-B of the IgG class. Mothers who are group A and B usually have IgM antibodies predominantly. In the UK, the disease is usually very mild; severe anaemia is uncommon and the child rarely requires treatment by exchange transfusion. Part of the difficulty in recognizing the disease is that the antiglobulin reaction carried out on the cord cells is usually negative or only very weakly positive. Two fairly consistent findings are an increase in osmotic fragility of the red cells and the presence of spherocytes in cord blood.

ABO HDN affects about one in 150 of all births. In certain parts of the world, however, ABO HDN is more common. In Jamaica, for instance, it is more frequent than HDN due to Rh-antibodies. This may in part result from the high concentrations of anti-A and anti-B in the population (Lindo-Haynes 1980).

MANAGEMENT OF MOTHER AND CHILD

It is vitally important to predict antenatally the birth of an affected infant so that labour can take place in a hospital equipped to carry out exchange transfusion within the first few hours of birth. Rh-negative mothers must therefore be examined for the presence of anti-D in their plasma during pregnancy. The ABO and Rh blood groups of all pregnant mothers are determined early in pregnancy, and all those who are Rh-negative are examined for the presence of anti-D at 12 weeks. Any anti-D present at this time was probably initiated during or soon after the previous pregnancy. A further examination is carried out at 28 weeks. This time is chosen because if anti-D is present, this is also the optimum time for carrying out amniocentesis for the antenatal determination of the severity of the disease.

A method of predicting the severity of the disease would be very valuable since a considerable proportion of affected infants are stillborn and about half of these deaths occur after the 36th week of pregnancy. Attempts at prediction take into account the amount of anti-D in the mother's plasma, the previous history of affected infants and examination of the bilirubin concentration in the amniotic fluid. None of these are reliable guides when taken singly, but prediction is improved when all three are considered together. Although there are many exceptions, on the whole there is a higher incidence of severe disease in children born to mothers who have high titres of anti-D (values over 256). As mentioned earlier, severe disease tends to run in families and a mother with one stillborn child has approximately a 70% chance of having a second stillbirth. Finally, estimation of the amount of bilirubin spectroscopically in the amniotic fluid at 28 weeks gives some, but by no means a reliable, indication of severity (Fairweather & Walker 1965) and indicates whether premature induction of labour should be carried out at a later date. Since about half the total number of stillbirths occur after the 36th week of pregnancy, induction at 36 weeks reduces the incidence of stillbirth.

As soon as the baby is born, cord blood must be obtained and the presence of antibody on the baby's red cells confirmed by the antiglobulin test. If this is positive (the strength of the reaction is no guide to severity) then haemoglobulin and plasma bilirubin concentration are estimated, using cord blood. It should be stressed that cord blood is of far greater value than either venous blood or skin-prick blood from the child, since the latter normally shows a rise in haemoglobin concentration from about 30 minutes after birth, due to transfer of blood from the placenta to baby before the cord is tied, followed by a subsequent fall in plasma volume. If the haemoglobin concentration is below the lower limit of normal of 13.5 g/dl an exchange transfusion with Rh-negative blood is required. If the haemoglobin concentration is within the normal range, the decision to give an immediate exchange transfusion rests on the bilirubin concentration. Some pediatricians perform an exchange transfusion if this is above 70 μmol/l but others have different criteria. Even if the cord haemoglobin concentration is normal, death can still occur from kernicterus if the ability to excrete bilirubin is poorly developed. About half the patients with haemoglobin concentrations within the normal range require an exchange transfusion because of a high bilirubin concentration.

The aims of exchange-transfusion are thus twofold. First, to replace the Rh-positive blood of the child with Rh-negative blood which does not react with anti-D and will thus survive normally. In those relatively rare cases where the antibody concerned is anti-c or anti-E, then blood lacking these antigens is used. Secondly, to prevent the bilirubin concentration rising to a value of 350 μmol/l, since kernicterus usually develops if this level is exceeded. Frequent estimations of bilirubin concentration are therefore necessary and several exchange-transfusions may be required.

PREVENTION OF RH IMMUNIZATION

It is now possible to bring about a very considerable reduction in the incidence of Rh immunization by the injection of anti-D into an Rh-negative mother within 36 hours of giving birth to an Rh-positive child. The injected anti-D combines with the fetal red cells in the mother's circulation and brings about their destruction in the spleen. The precise mechanism by which the suppression of immunization is brought about is not known, but it is assumed that splenic destruction of fetal red cells must divert D antigen on the surface of the cells away from those sites in the immunological system where antibody production is initiated.

Two observations led to the use of anti-D in the prevention of Rh immunization. First, it was known that anti-D only occasionally developed in the mother if the baby was group A and the mother group O. The suggested explanation of this phenomenon was that the maternal anti-A reacted with the group A fetal red cells and led to their immediate destruction, thus preventing the cells from immunizing the mothers. It was thought that if anti-A could reduce the incidence of immunization, then anti-D might have the same effect. Trials with male volunteers given Rh-positive cells and with women with more than 0.1 ml of fetal cells in their circulation showed that the administration of anti-D would suppress active anti-D production (Clarke 1967, 1968). Secondly, there was an early immunological observation made by Smith in 1909 and since confirmed many times, that if an antigen is mixed with its specific antibody and injected into an animal, the antibody response of that animal to the antigen is considerably reduced compared to that seen when the antigen alone is injected. This led a group in New York (Freda et al. 1967) independently to carry out trials with anti-D, which were also successful. The injection of anti-D has been shown not only to prevent the appearance of anti-D in the mother 6 months after labour, but also to prevent its appearance during a subsequent pregnancy with an Rh-positive child.

The effectiveness of the treatment will depend partly on the dose of anti-D that is injected. Since the anti-D acts by diverting fetal cells away from stimulating the immunological system, it is reasonable to suppose that the larger the dose, the more effective it will be, especially when the transplacental bleed is a large one. The dose of anti-D that is being used at the moment is 100–300 μg, and there is some evidence that this may protect against a transplacental bleed of 5–15 ml of whole blood. However, it is known that this dose is inadequate against a bleed of 50 ml or more (Dudok de Wit et al. 1968) and thus larger doses of anti-D must be given when it is known that the transplacental passage of blood is of this order. In order to detect these large transplacental bleeds, it is necessary to estimate the number of fetal cells in the maternal circulation by the acid-elution technique.

Prophylaxis with anti-D has now been used for a sufficient time to assess its effectiveness. It would appear that the incidence of HDN in the second Rh-positive child born to a mother who had been treated with anti-D is about 0.5–1%. This figure is to be compared to an incidence of about 17% in untreated women. The failures in preventive therapy are mainly due either to the transplacental passage at labour of large amounts of fetal red cells (25–50 ml or more) which would not be covered by the standard dose of 100–300 μg of anti-D, or they may be due to primary immunization early in the course of the first pregnancy. The frequency of immunization occurring in primigravidae can be considerably reduced by the injection of anti-D at 28 weeks of pregnancy. The combination of anti-D given at 28 weeks and post-partum can be extremely effective, as has been demonstrated in Manitoba, where all women at risk within the state are treated in this way. The protection rate is over 98%, with the result that perinatal deaths due to HDN have been reduced from about 20 per year to about 1 every 6 years (Bowman & Pollock 1983).

It is also possible to prevent the production of anti-D when a large amount of Rh-positive blood has been inadvertently transfused, the dose of anti-D being of the order of 20 µg for each ml of red cells transfused.

OBJECTIVES IN LEARNING

1 To know the cause of HDN, the antigens concerned, the mechanism of immunization and the approximate risk to a mother of becoming immunized.

2 To know the principles of antenatal care concerned with predicting both the presence and severity of the disease.

3 To know the clinical features and extent of variation in severity of HDN, and the causes of disability and death.

4 To know the method of assessment of the severity in the infant immediately after birth and the indications for exchange transfusions.

REFERENCES

Bowman J.M. & Pollack J. (1983) Rh immunization in Manitoba: progress in prevention and management. *Can. Med. Assoc. J.*, **129**: 343.

Clarke C.A. (1967) Prevention of Rh-haemolytic disease. *Br. Med. J.*, **4**: 7.

Clarke C.A. (1968) Prevention of Rhesus iso-immunization. *Lancet*, **ii**, 1.

Dudok de Wit C., Borst-Eilers E., Weerdt Ch. M.V.D., & Kloosterman G.J. (1968) Prevention of Rhesus Immunization. A controlled clinical trial with a comparatively low dose of anti-D immunoglobulin. *Br. Med. J.*, **4**: 477.

Fairweather D.V.I., Walker W. (1965) Current views on the management of rhesus isoimmunization. *Ob. Gynecol. Digest.*, **7**; 49.

Freda V.J., Gorman J.G., Pollack W., Robertson J.G., Jennings E.A., Sullivan J.F. (1967) Prevention of Rh isoimmunization. *J. Am. Med. Ass.*, **199**: 390.

Giblett E.R. (1964) Blood-group antibodies causing haemolytic disease of the newborn. *Clin. Obstet. Gynec.*, **7**: 1044.

Levine P., Burnham L., Katzin E.M., Vogel P. (1941) The role of isoimmunization in the pathogenesis of erythroblastosis foetalis. *Am. J. Obstet. Gynec.*, **42**: 925.

Lindo-Haynes G. (1980) Blood group distribution of ABO haemolytic disease of the newborn in Jamaica. *Med. Lab. Sci.*, **37**: 263.

Chapter 5
Iron Metabolism, Iron Deficiency Anaemia and other Hypochromic Microcytic Anaemias

METABOLISM OF IRON

Distribution of iron in the body

Essential iron-containing compounds are found in the plasma and in all cells. Since ionized iron is toxic, iron is always present within the haem moiety of a haemoprotein (e.g. haemoglobin, myoglobin and cytochrome) or directly bound to a protein (e.g. transferrin, ferritin and haemosiderin). The total body iron content of a healthy adult varies between 2 and 5 g. About two-thirds of this iron is found in the haemoglobin of red cells: since 1 ml of red cells contains approximately 1 mg of iron, an adult has about 2 g of iron in the red cell mass. About 0.15 g of iron is present in the myoglobin of muscle cells and in the respiratory enzymes of all cells. Most of the remainder of the iron is stored in the macrophages of the spleen and bone marrow and in both the Kupffer and parenchymal cells of the liver. The stores of iron vary from 0 to 1 g or more. Storage iron exists in the two forms, ferritin and haemosiderin. Ferritin is composed of a protein shell and encloses an iron core containing up to 4500 atoms of iron. Haemosiderin is composed of aggregates of ferritin molecules which have partly lost their protein shell. Ferritin is water soluble and is thus not seen on ordinary histological sections as it is removed during the preparation of the slide. Haemosiderin, on the other hand, can be seen as golden-brown granules in unstained preparations or as blue granules inside macrophages when stained by Perls' acid ferrocyanide method (Prussian Blue reaction). When the total body stores change, the two forms of storage iron increase or decrease together.

Dynamic state of body iron

Iron is continuously circulating through the plasma bound to the protein, transferrin. The major part of this circulating iron is derived from the daily destruction of approximately 20 ml of red cells, which liberates 20 mg of iron. There is also a further 10–15 mg of iron carried through the plasma daily. This iron is derived from the iron stores and from absorption in the gastrointestinal tract. Plasma iron is rapidly removed mainly by erythropoietic tissue in the bone marrow but part goes to other dividing cells and to the iron stores. The half-time for passage of iron through the circulation is approximately 100 minutes.

Iron absorption

An average diet contains approximately 10–20 mg of iron per day, mostly in organic form but there is some in inorganic form. Iron is widely distributed and is present in both vegetables and meat, the concentration being higher in the latter. Adults who have normal iron stores absorb approximately 5–10% of their total intake, i.e. they absorb 0.5–2 mg/day. The precise amount absorbed is dependent on the chemical form of iron in the food. Iron in the form of haem is absorbed best. The haem molecule is taken up by intestinal epithelial cells within which the iron is split from the porphyrin ring. Non-haem iron is less well absorbed as it can be readily bound and made non-absorbable by ligands such as phytate and phosphate that are found in food. Ferric iron must be reduced to the ferrous form before absorption; hence oral iron is given therapeutically as the ferrous salt. Ascorbic acid promotes the absorption of non-haem iron, partly because it is a reducing agent and partly because it forms a molecular complex with it, which is readily absorbed. Iron is absorbed in the upper half of the small intestine.

It has long been established that the prevalence of gastric atrophy and of achlorhydria is higher in patients with iron-deficiency anaemia than in healthy people, but there has been a great deal of argument as to the relationship between the gastric changes and the iron deficiency. The most probable relationship is that the gastric atrophy is the primary event and that the consequent achlorhydria is an aetiological factor in the development of iron deficiency. In most instances the gastric mucosa does not return to normal after cure of the iron deficiency. Moreover, Goldberg et al. (1963) found that ^{59}FeCl$_3$ is less well absorbed in iron-deficient patients with achlorhydria (18% absorption) than in those who secrete HCl (57% absorption), suggesting that HCl promotes the absorption of inorganic iron.

Absorption of iron does not remain constant at 5–10% of total intake but is altered according to both the state of iron stores and the rate of erythropoiesis. When iron intake is in excess of that required for growth and to replenish the daily loss of iron from the body, iron is stored in the liver, spleen and bone marrow. As iron stores increase, the rate of accumulation in the stores decreases, mainly due to a slowing in the rate of absorption and partly due to increased loss as the result of an increase in iron content of cells shed from the body. Eventually an equilibrium is reached when iron stores remain constant. The upper limit of normal iron stores in healthy people is about 1 g. On the other hand, when iron stores decrease, the absorptive mechanism is stimulated and the percentage of iron absorbed is increased so that, in iron deficiency, absorption may rise to over 50% of total intake.

Iron that enters from the gut contents into the epithelial cells is either passed on to the plasma transferrin or remains within the cells and combines with apoferritin to form ferritin. The transfer of iron from the epithelial cells into the plasma is controlled by an unidentified mechanism which responds to iron requirements, the rate being rapid when stores are reduced or the rate of erythropoiesis is increased. Iron not transferred to the plasma remains in the epithelial cells until desquamation takes place and the iron is then excreted in the faeces. See Aisen (1982) for a review of iron absorption.

Iron loss

There is no specific excretory mechanism for iron. Nevertheless, there is an inevitable daily loss of iron as a result of the continuous exfoliation of gut and skin epithelial cells, all of which have iron-containing enzymes. In adults, this loss is approximately 0.6 mg/day (Finch & Loden 1959). The extra loss in women due to menstruation and pregnancy is discussed later (p. 66).

IRON-DEPLETION AND IRON-DEFICIENCY ANAEMIA

As body iron stores are depleted, two phases can be recognized. The first stage is *iron depletion without anaemia*, when stores are exhausted but the haemoglobin concentration is either unaffected or falls only slightly so that, although it is slightly below the normal for that individual, it is still within the generally accepted normal range as defined by the World Health Organization (WHO) criteria (p. 15). Further depletion of body iron results in an insufficient amount of iron being present to maintain the red-cell mass; haemoglobin concentration then falls below the normal range and *iron-deficiency anaemia* results.

In any given population, there are approximately equal numbers of people with iron depletion alone and with iron-deficiency anaemia. It is probable that the course of events in the development of iron depletion without and with anaemia is as follows. An individual with some iron stores may be in iron equilibrium by absorbing, say, 10% of the iron in the diet. If a negative iron balance occurs as a result of chronic haemorrhage, iron stores will diminish and by the time they are finally depleted, iron absorption may have increased to a value which brings the individual back into iron balance, but without iron stores. This state would then be maintained until the equilibrium was altered again. For instance, if the rate of iron loss increased still further so that it exceeded the rate at which it could be absorbed from the diet, then anaemia would ensue. On the other hand, if iron loss decreased, then iron would start to accumulate in the stores again, but this would lead to reduced absorption and a new equilibrium would be reached.

Prevalence of iron deficiency

Iron-deficiency anaemia appears most frequently during two periods of life; namely, in infants of both sexes and in women during the child-bearing period.

Prevalence of iron deficiency in infancy

Iron deficiency is frequently found between the ages of 6 months and 5 years, the highest prevalence being at about 12 months. Davis *et al.* (1960) concluded that about half of a group of West Indian infants and one-quarter of European infants living in London had iron deficiency, as judged by the finding of a mean cell haemoglobin concentration (MCHC) of below 30 g/dl. After the age of 3 years, iron deficiency is less common but not insignificant. Among people of modest income in the USA, approximately 5% of the children aged 5–11 years had iron-deficiency anaemia and a further 10% had iron depletion without anaemia (Cook *et al.* 1976).

Prevalence of iron deficiency in adolescents and adults

The prevalence of iron deficiency has always been found to be much higher in women than in men, especially during the fertile years. Thus, Jacobs *et al.* (1969) investigated a random sample of adult women in Wales and found that

12% of the women had iron depletion alone and 10% of the women also had iron-deficiency anaemia. In a study in both Latin America and in the North Western USA, approximately 10% of women were iron depleted and a further 10% were also anaemic (Cook et al. 1971; Cook et al. 1976).

The prevalence of iron deficiency in males is much lower. In a sample from Wales, 4.5% had iron depletion and 1.5% were also anaemic (Jacobs et al. 1969). Brumfitt (1960) found an incidence of approximately 1% in 17–21-year-old male recruits for the Royal Army Medical Corps. Elwood et al. (1964b) found the prevalence of iron-deficiency anaemia for 14-year-old school children in Cardiff to be 2.4% for boys and 4.2% for girls.

Fry (1961) investigated the prevalence of iron-deficiency anaemia in general practice and found that most males presented with iron deficiency before the age of 10, or after 50 years. By contrast, the peak periods of presentation in women was during and immediately after the child-bearing period (30–50 years).

Giles and Burton (1960) found that 66% of pregnant women had haemoglobin concentrations below 11.8 g/dl when first seen in the antenatal clinic. Based on the response to iron therapy it was concluded that the majority of these women were iron deficient, although folic acid deficiency and haemodilution (p. 15) were also aetiological factors in the anaemia.

Causes of iron deficiency

Iron stores become depleted when the rate of absorption of iron is insufficient to replace iron lost from the body. Inadequate absorption may be due to a low iron content of the diet or to impairment of intestinal absorptive mechanisms. On the other hand, loss of iron usually through haemorrhage may occur at a greater rate than replacement from a normal diet by a normal absorptive mechanism. The causes of iron deficiency are summarized in Table 5.1.

Abnormal uterine bleeding and pregnancy are common causes of iron deficiency. Amongst the other causes, an inadequate diet and diseases of the gastrointestinal tract predominate. In a retrospective review of 378 in-patients with iron deficiency by Beveridge et al. (1965), 19% were found to be due to a poor diet. Gastrointestinal bleeding due to various causes accounted for about 40% and gastrectomy and steatorrhoea accounted for a further 14% of cases.

Gastrectomy is frequently followed by iron deficiency: Tovey and Clark (1980) found that 40% of patients were anaemic 9–14 years after a partial gastrectomy and that 53% relapsed after one course of iron therapy. Iron deficiency in these patients is due to inadequate absorption but the cause of the latter is not certain. The most likely explanation is the rapid rate of passage of food through the upper part of the small intestine that is known to occur following gastrectomy. As iron is absorbed in the jejunum, the rapid passage reduces the time available for release of iron from food protein and its subsequent absorption. Bleeding from the mucosal remnant of the stomach has also been observed, sometimes at a rate of over 150 ml of blood per month (Holt et al. 1970).

The malabsorption syndrome (e.g. due to coeliac disease) also frequently causes iron deficiency and iron-deficiency anaemia.

Table 5.1 Causes of iron deficiency.

Reduced iron stores at birth due to prematurity

Inadequate intake (prolonged breast or bottle feeding without iron supplementation, vegetarian diets, poverty)

Increased requirement (pregnancy and lactation)

Chronic haemorrhage
  Uterine (menorrhagia, metrorrhagia)
  Gastrointestinal (e.g. hiatus hernia, oesophageal
    varices, peptic ulceration, Meckel's diverticulum,
    colonic diverticulosis, ulcerative colitis,
    carcinoma of the stomach, colon or rectum,
    haemorrhoids, hereditary telangiectasia—see p. 160,
    hookworm infestation*)
  Other (e.g. self-inflicted, recurrent haematuria)

Malabsorption (coeliac disease, partial gastrectomy)

Chronic intravascular haemolysis leading to haemoglobinuria and
  haemosiderinuria (rare)

*This is a very common cause of iron deficiency in tropical countries.

Causes of iron deficiency in infancy

There are two factors which predispose to iron deficiency in infancy; namely, inadequate iron stores at birth and inadequate amount of iron in the diet. As about half the iron stores are deposited in the last month of fetal life, premature babies may deplete their iron stores before starting on iron-rich solid food. The growing child needs to absorb 0.5–0.9 mg of iron each day during the first year (Burman 1982); this cannot be supplied by either human or cow's milk, since both sources have low concentrations of iron and 5–9 pints would be required to provide sufficient iron for the child's daily needs.

A 4 kg baby is provided with sufficient iron stores to last for 6 months. It is thus important that the baby should be started on iron-rich foods by this time. On the other hand, a 2.5 kg baby has only sufficient iron to grow to 4 or 5 kg, which occurs before solid food is given and hence liquid iron supplements must be provided.

Inadequate iron intake may continue once solid food has been started. It is for this reason that specially prepared infant foods, such as those based on cereals, have an artificially raised iron content. It is thought that about 10 mg of iron per day is required in the diet during the first 2 years of life; a substantial proportion of infants in this age group in the British population receives less than 10 mg of iron in their daily diet at the present time.

Causes of iron deficiency in adult females

Since the prevalence of iron deficiency is so much higher in women than in men, it is reasonable to assign the cause to excessive loss of iron through menstruation and child bearing, and this assumption is supported by the available evidence.

Two reports may be cited. First, that of Scott & Pritchard (1967) who investigated 114 college women aged 19–25 years in Texas. One-quarter of the women had no demonstrable iron stores in the marrow, about two-thirds of the women had iron stores of less than 350 mg, and only 5% had sufficient stainable marrow iron to suggest that the stores were in the range of 500–1000 mg, which is the generally accepted level for normal iron stores.

Secondly, the measurement of blood loss during menstruation shows that the rate of loss in many women is sufficient to reduce the iron stores rapidly. Halberg *et al.* (1966) studied women working in a factory and found the mean loss of blood was 34 ml (range 2–200 ml) with each period. He considered that this might underestimate the loss in the population as a whole, which may be as high as an average of 43 ml in each period. The group of women losing more than 60 ml with each period showed a reduction in haemoglobin concentration and MCHC, a fall in plasma iron concentration and a rise in total iron-binding capacity compared to those losing smaller amounts. These findings suggest that many women losing 60 ml or more are depleted of iron stores (Fig. 5.1). Ten of the 137 women had iron-deficiency anaemia (haemoglobin concentration less than 12 g/dl) and the average menstrual loss of these iron-deficient women, 58 ml, was considerably higher than the mean for the group as a whole. The diagram shown in Fig. 5.2 taken from Jacobs *et al.* (1965) shows the monthly menstrual loss and the iron requirements in 151 normal women. The daily iron requirements are based on a value of 10% iron absorption from the diet, and it can be seen that women losing 80 ml of blood or more require 21 mg of iron or over as a daily intake, i.e. more than is present in a normal diet.

Iron deficiency in pregnancy

Haemoglobin concentration falls in pregnancy and normal lower limits have been variously reported to be between 10 and 12 g/dl; the WHO has recommended that a lower limit of normal of 11 g/dl should be taken for practical purposes. The main reason for this fall is an increase in plasma volume; red-cell mass increases by 200–500 ml but there is an even greater increase in plasma volume resulting in haemodilution. The increase in red-cell mass requires an extra 200–500 mg of iron but this is offset by the fact that there is a reduction in iron loss by approximately the same amount due to amenorrhoea.

The total amount of iron required by the mother during each pregnancy is high, being of the order of 500–700 mg. The fetus requires approximately 250 mg and the rest is lost in the placenta and through haemorrhage; the average amount of blood lost during parturition has been estimated to be of the order of 300 ml (Newton *et al.* 1961). Thus, pregnant women are required to absorb each day about 2–3 mg more than men, in whom the basic requirement is about 0.6 mg/day. This is more than can be absorbed from a normal unsupplemented diet and unless the mother starts pregnancy with more than about 200 mg of storage iron, iron depletion will almost certainly occur.

As a group, women of child-bearing age have lower iron stores than men of a similar age, and it is possible that only those women who have a high iron intake and have had small menstrual losses are able to maintain adequate iron stores during pregnancy. This is reflected in two findings: first, that of Foulkes

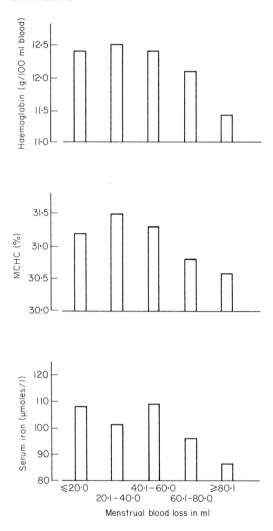

Fig. 5.1   Mean values of haemoglobin concentration, MCHC and serum iron concentration in relation to menstrual blood loss. Redrawn from Halberg *et al.* (1966).

and Goldie (1982) that 87% of women whose serum ferritin levels were below 50 μg/ml in early pregnancy became anaemic later unless iron supplements were given; second, that of Chanarin and Rothman (1965) who examined 49 marrow biopsies from women towards the end of pregnancy, including 16 women who had normal haematological values. Only four of the patients had demonstrable iron stores, and all of these were on iron supplements during pregnancy.

Clinical presentation

Symptoms

Iron-deficiency anaemia develops slowly, thereby permitting various adaptive mechanisms to operate and compensate for the effects of the developing

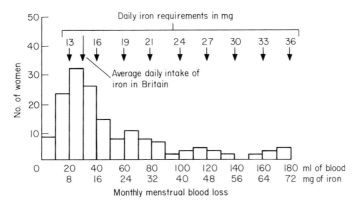

Fig. 5.2 Menstrual blood loss in 151 normal women. The daily iron requirements are calculated on the basis that 10% of the iron in the diet is absorbed. Adapted from Jacobs *et al.* (1965).

anaemia (p. 16). Symptoms attributable to anaemia (p. 16) are, therefore, only seen when the haemoglobin falls below about 8 g/dl. Various symptoms referable to the cardiovascular and nervous system such as malaise, fatigue, faintness, lack of concentration, dizziness, irritability, headache, palpitations, breathlessness, swelling of ankles and pain in the chest, are reported by some patients with haemoglobin values between 8 and 12 g/dl. However, these symptoms can clearly be caused by a great variety of other diseases and are common in neurosis. Berry & Nash (1954) have shown that this type of symptom is common in people without anaemia and conversely many people with anaemia do not have symptoms. Berry & Nash found that the prevalence of anaemia (Hb 10–12 g/dl) in women who stated that they were fit and were not tired or breathless was the same (13.8% of them were anaemic) as the prevalence in those who complained that they were not fit and were always tired and breathless (12.9% anaemic).

Peculiar dietary cravings (pica), e.g. for soil or ice, may be found in some cases of iron-deficiency anaemia.

Dysphagia and iron deficiency

For many years the symptom of post-cricoid dysphagia, associated in some cases with a web or stricture, has been linked with a hypochromic anaemia and the presence of the two together has been known as the Paterson–Kelly syndrome. Since the hypochromic anaemia was due to iron deficiency, it came to be generally held that the iron deficiency was the cause of the epithelial changes leading to dysphagia. Some evidence suggests that this may not be so (Jacobs & Kilpatrick 1964). Elwood *et al.* (1964a) studied the prevalence of post-cricoid dysphagia in people living in the Rhondda Fach, Wales, and found dysphagia in 1% of males and 5% of females over the age of 45 years. To their surprise, the prevalence of anaemia and of iron deficiency in those patients with dysphagia was the same as in carefully matched control patients without dysphagia, suggesting that iron deficiency may not be an aetiological factor. Nevertheless, about half the patients who have a sufficiently severe dysphagia to warrant hospital admission have hypochromic anaemia with low serum iron levels (Jacobs & Kilpatrick 1964). Thus, present evidence suggests that iron deficiency may not be an aetiological factor in post-cricoid dysphagia. When it is present it seems to be secondary either to the reduction in food intake resulting from the dysphagia, or to the achlorhydria which is frequently found in this condition.

Signs

The signs of anaemia are discussed on p. 16. Beveridge *et al.* (1965) reported the signs associated with a deficiency of iron in epithelial tissues and their prevalence to be: redness of the tongue and loss of papillae (glossitis), 39%; abnormal nails, either spoon-shaped (koilonychia) or flat, 28%; angular stomatitis, 14%. These signs are much less frequently seen today than in the past. The tip of the spleen is palpable in about 10% of cases.

Haematological changes

If iron loss continues after body stores are depleted, then there is insufficient iron to maintain a normal total red-cell mass and the haemoglobin concentration falls. There is a progression of changes in the peripheral blood (see p. 202 for methods of estimation). Patients with mild anaemia may initially have a normal mean cell volume (MCV) and mean corpuscular haemoglobin (MCH) with anisocytosis of red cells. Soon the red cells become microcytic, as shown by a fall in the MCV and this is accompanied by a similar fall in the MCH. The concentration of haemoglobin in each cell (MCHC) is thus unchanged initially. It is only in the later stages that the MCHC is reduced. This is exemplified by the

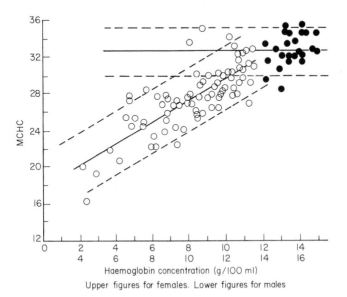

Fig. 5.3 The relationship between MCHC and the haemoglobin concentration in 80 iron deficient (○) and 25 normal (●) subjects. Redrawn from Beutler (1959).

observations of Beutler (1959) that 19 out of 80 patients with iron-deficiency anaemia had an MCHC within the normal range of 30–35 g/dl. It was only when the haemoglobin concentration fell below 7 g/dl in women and 9 g/dl in men that the MCHC always fell below the normal range (Fig. 5.3).

On examination of a peripheral blood film, many patients are found to have red cells with hypochromia (p. 18), a reduced diameter (microcytosis) and increased variation in size (anisocytosis) and shape (poikilocytosis) (Fig. 5.4) Some target cells may also be present.

A marrow smear stained by Perls' acid ferrocyanide method shows an absence of stainable iron in the macrophages within the bone marrow fragments (Plates 9, 10). Occasionally, traces of stainable iron may be found. Erythropoiesis is normoblastic.

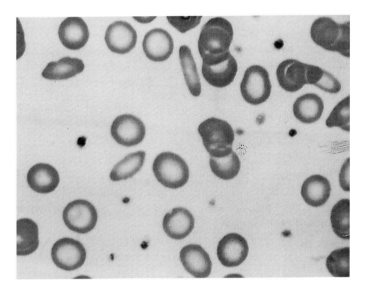

Fig. 5.4 Peripheral blood film from a patient with untreated iron deficiency anaemia. Hypochromic microcytes and elongated ('pencil-shaped') poikilocytes are present.

Serum iron

There is a wide diurnal variation in the normal values for serum iron. The average value is 21 μmol/l, but the values may vary from 50 μmol/l in the morning to 10 μmol/l in the evening (Hamilton *et al.* 1950). Women show a pronounced fall during menstruation; at this time serum iron levels may be as low as 3.5 μmol/l (Zilva & Patston 1966). However, when the haemoglobin concentration falls below 9 g/dl in iron deficiency, the diurnal variation is less and the serum-iron concentration is usually consistently below 10 μmol/l (Beutler *et al.* 1958).

Total iron-binding capacity (TIBC) and transferrin saturation

The total amount of iron that can be bound to plasma transferrin is usually in the range of 50–70 μmol/l plasma. In iron-deficiency anaemia the iron-binding capacity is invariably raised when the haemoglobin concentration falls below 9 g/dl and is often raised when the haemoglobin is in the range of 9–11 g/dl. Thus, a raised TIBC is a useful diagnostic criterion, although the finding of raised levels in those taking oral contraceptives reduces its value considerably. TIBC is frequently reduced below normal in patients with infections, neoplasms and rheumatoid arthritis and thus helps to distinguish anaemia in these diseases from that due to iron deficiency (Bainton & Finch 1964).

The percentage of transferrin that is bound with iron (i.e. the ratio of serum iron concentration to total iron-binding capacity expressed as a percentage) is a very useful index for the diagnosis of iron depletion. It has been found that a value of 16% or lower for the transferrin saturation indicates lack of iron stores.

Serum ferritin levels

Ferritin is an iron storage protein. It is found in many cell types but especially in the macrophages of the liver, spleen and bone marrow and in hepatocytes. It is also found in very low concentrations in the serum. Sensitive immunological assays have now been developed for assessing serum ferritin levels and it has been shown that there is a direct relationship between serum ferritin levels and the amount of iron stored in the marrow (Walters *et al.* 1973). Although this test is more complicated to carry out than serum iron and transferrin saturation assays, it is superior to these tests in differentiating the anaemia resulting from iron deficiency from that due to chronic disease. Each 1 µg/l of ferritin in the plasma indicates that there are about 10 mg of stored iron in the liver. Thus, a plasma level of 100 µg/l represents a store of 1000 mg of iron. In the absence of iron stores, the plasma ferritin level is less than 12 µg/l.

Even serum ferritin levels are not a completely reliable guide to the quantity of storage iron. Sometimes patients are found with serum ferritin levels above 12 µg/l but who have no stainable iron in bone marrow aspirates. This is usually due to co-existent acute and chronic infections or malignancies, which raise serum ferritin levels above that expected from the amount of storage iron.

Measurement of iron absorption

Some patients who are diagnosed as having iron deficiency do not respond to adequate therapy with oral iron. In such patients, it may be necessary to measure iron absorption, by giving a small standard dose of radioactive ferric chloride (^{59}Fe) to a fasting patient and measuring excretion in the faeces. The amount absorbed is the difference between intake and excretion. Normally the amount absorbed under these conditions is in the range 5–30%. This value is higher than the percentage absorption of iron present in food since, in the radioactive test, the iron is provided in a readily absorbable soluble form and the patient is fasting, whereas the iron in food is combined to protein and is thus not so readily available for absorption.

In iron deficiency, iron absorption is stimulated and the amount absorbed is usually above 50%. Patients who are found to have an iron-deficiency anaemia but who have not responded by increasing iron absorption (i.e. iron absorption remains at less than 10% when measured by one of the radioactive techniques), probably have intestinal malabsorption (Badenoch & Callender 1960).

Diagnosis of iron depletion without anaemia

Iron depletion without anaemia can be defined as a state in which there is biochemical evidence of iron lack but haemoglobin concentrations are within the normal limits. If an appropriately stained marrow smear is examined, iron stores will be absent or virtually absent. The biochemical evidence usually consists of: a decreased serum iron level and an increased total iron-binding capacity (i.e. a low transferrin saturation); a low plasma ferritin; and an increase in red-cell protoporphyrin (Table 5.2). As has been emphasized, none of these tests is completely reliable, especially single serum iron measurements, but the probability of detecting iron depletion increases with the number of investigations that yield positive results.

Although the haemoglobin concentration of a patient with depleted iron stores may be within the generally accepted normal range, the value may be below the normal value for that person when iron stores are adequate. To illustrate this, Garby et al. (1969) gave iron supplements to a group of apparently normal women and found that a substantial number whose PCV was above the accepted lower limit of 0.35 showed a rise in PCV (Fig. 5.5).

Treatment of iron-deficiency anaemia

Treatment should start with the oral administration of 200 mg anhydrous ferrous sulphate (containing 60 mg of elemental iron) three times daily, as this is the easiest, cheapest and safest method. Stevens (1958) found that the minimal response in iron-deficient patients was a rise in haemoglobin concentration of 2 g/dl in 3 weeks (Fig. 5.6) and most had rises in excess of this. The haemoglobin concentration of the patient should therefore be measured again 3 weeks later to determine whether there has been an adequate response. If the patient has not responded the following should be considered:

1   That the patient has not taken the tablets. About one-third of antenatal patients in hospital and general practice were found not to be taking iron tablets which had been prescribed for them (Afifi et al. 1966). The authors pointed out that if this prevalence held throughout the country, then this would represent a

Table 5.2   Measurements of iron status in normal people, individuals with iron depletion without anaemia and in iron deficiency anaemia.

	Normal	Iron depletion without anaemia	Iron deficiency anaemia
Serum iron	10–30 µmol/l	<10	<10
Total iron binding capacity	50–70 µmol/l	>70	>70
Transferrin saturation	>16%	<16%	<16%
Serum ferritin	12–150 µg/l	<12	<12
Hb concentration	Within normal range	Within normal range	Below normal range

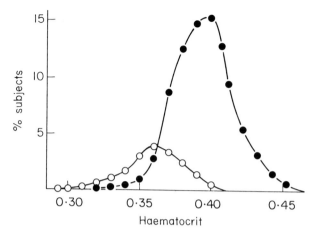

Fig. 5.5. Haematocrit values obtained from Swedish women before they took 60 mg of iron daily for 3 months. ●, women who showed no change in haematocrit. ○, women whose haematocrit increased in response to the iron therapy. Note that a substantial number of the women whose haematocrit was above the generally accepted lower limit or normal of 0.35 showed a response to iron therapy. Redrawn from Garby *et al.* (1969).

wastage of iron equivalent to eight small motor cars each year. One of the common reasons for not taking iron tablets is that the patient claims that they cause gastrointestinal symptoms, such as pain, diarrhoea or constipation. There is undoubtedly a psychological element in these symptoms. Girdwood (1952) found that side-effects caused by ferrous sulphate given as green pills disappeared when white ferrous sulphate pills were substituted. Those patients who cannot tolerate ferrous sulphate, whatever the cause, should be given another absorbable iron compound (e.g. ferrous gluconate, etc.).

2   That the patient has the malabsorption syndrome. Patients with this syndrome often present with iron-deficiency anaemia.

3   If the iron deficiency was due to haemorrhage, this may still be operative, e.g. continued bleeding from the gut.

4   That the initial diagnosis was incorrect, or that B_{12} or folate deficiency is also present.

The purpose of treatment with iron is not only to restore the total red-cell volume to normal but also to replenish iron stores. The former is easy but the latter is difficult. If the patient absorbs only 10% of the 180 mg iron ingested each day as ferrous sulphate, then it will take approximately 2 months to raise iron stores to about 1 g. In practice it has been found that the percentage of iron absorbed is often less than this and the patient should therefore be persuaded to continue taking iron for 4–6 months after the haemoglobin level becomes normal.

Patients with a gastrectomy relapse so frequently after a single course of iron that it has been recommended that they should be given daily continuous therapy with 200 mg ferrous sulphate a day (Tovey & Clark 1980).

Patients with the malabsorption syndrome and those who cannot tolerate any

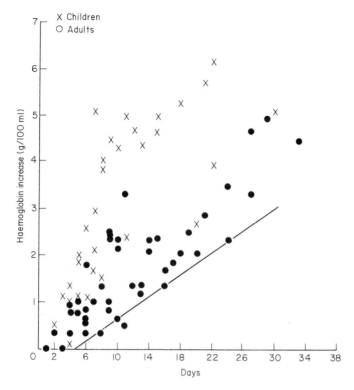

Fig. 5.6 Blood regeneration following intramuscular iron therapy. The minimal response of iron-deficient patients is indicated as a straight line intersecting 2 g/100 ml haemoglobin increase at 21 days. Children responded much faster than adults. Provided the iron is absorbed, oral iron produces as rapid a response as intramuscular iron. Redrawn from Stevens (1958).

form of iron orally, should be given iron parenterally. Usually, iron dextran (Imferon) or iron sorbitol (Jectofer) is given daily by deep intramuscular injection, in a 10-day course. The total dose can be calculated approximately from the extent of the anaemia. Thus, a patient with a haemoglobin concentration of 7 g/dl will have a red-cell volume of 1000 ml (half the normal value). That is to say, 1000 mg of iron must be given to restore the red-cell volume (1 ml cells contains 1 mg iron), and a further 1000 mg are given to restore iron stores.

The intramuscular preparations, such as iron-dextran, contain iron bound to a carbohydrate compound. The iron-carbohydrate complex does not ionize and is, therefore, relatively non-toxic. The complexes reach the circulation and are removed and slowly degraded by macrophages. The free iron resulting from this degradation is released extracellularly and thus becomes available for uptake into cells. The rate of rise in haemoglobin concentration is not faster with parenteral iron than with oral iron, so that parenteral iron should not be given in the hope of obtaining a quick response.

The total amount of iron required for treatment can be given as iron-dextran intravenously, diluted in a large volume of saline and infused over 8–10 hours.

Systemic reactions, such as headache, fever, nausea and joint pains are common and serious hypersensitivity reactions occur rarely.

It has been stated (p. 68) that iron stores are usually absent in pregnancy, but there is controversy as to whether all pregnant women should be treated with iron irrespective of their haemoglobin concentration or only when the haemoglobin falls below an arbitrary value (such as 11.0 g/dl, p. 67). The argument against treating all pregnant women with iron is that when this is done, haematological investigations are often omitted, so that other causes of anaemia (such as folate deficiency) are missed. Moreover, a considerable proportion of patients do not take the prescribed tablets, nor is the obstetrician informed of this. Some are of the opinion that it is safest to estimate the haemoglobin concentration frequently and prescribe iron when required (Verloop 1970).

OTHER HYPOCHROMIC MICROCYTIC ANAEMIAS

Hypochromic microcytic red cells are formed when there is a substantial impairment of the synthesis of the haem moiety or of the α- or β-globin chains of the haemoglobin molecule. Iron deficiency is the most common cause of these changes; some of the other causes are listed in Table 5.3. Table 5.4 shows the way in which the three most common causes of hypochromia and microcytosis can be distinguished from each other on the basis of the serum iron level, the total iron-binding capacity (TIBC), serum ferritin level and the quantity of stainable iron within bone marrow macrophages.

Anaemia of chronic disorders

A common type of anaemia seen in hospital inpatients is that associated with chronic disorders such as chronic infections (e.g. tuberculosis), neoplasia and

Table 5.3 Some causes of hypochromic microcytic red cells.

Iron deficiency[1]

Anaemia of chronic disorders[1,3] (p. 77)

Sideroblastic anaemias[1]

Lead poisoning[1]

Heterozygosity and
  homozygosity for β-thalassaemia[2] (p. 45)

α^+-thalassaemia trait[2,3](p. 43)

α^0-thalassaemia trait[2] (p. 44)

HbH disease[2] (p. 44)

Heterozygotes and homozygotes
  for HbE[2] (p. 37)

Homozygotes for HbC[2,3] (p. 37)

1 The hypochromia is caused by impaired haem synthesis
2 The hypochromia is caused by impaired globin chain synthesis
3 Some patients have normochromic normocytic red cells

Table 5.4 Investigations useful in distinguishing between three important causes of hypochromic microcytes.

Investigation	Iron deficiency anaemia	Anaemia of chronic disorders	Thalassaemia trait
Serum iron	Low	Low	Normal
TIBC	Increased or normal	Decreased or normal	Normal
Serum ferritin	Decreased	Normal or increased	Normal
Marrow iron stores	Markedly decreased or absent	Normal or increased	Normal or increased

rheumatoid arthritis. The characteristic findings are as follows:

1   A mild or, occasionally, moderate degree of anaemia; the red cells are commonly normochromic and normocytic but may be hypochromic and microcytic.

2   A low serum iron concentration, a normal or low total iron-binding capacity (TIBC), a reduced transferrin saturation and a normal or increased serum ferritin; iron stores are present in the marrow and may be increased.

The anaemia usually develops within the first 2 months of the disease and then stabilizes at a fairly constant level. The anaemia must be distinguished from that seen in iron deficiency, since it does not respond to iron therapy. The differential diagnosis could be reliably made by studying the iron stores in the marrow: stainable macrophage iron is absent or virtually absent in iron deficiency and normal or increased in chronic disorders. However, the diagnosis can usually be made without marrow aspiration on the basis of the results of the serum iron level, TIBC and serum ferritin level (Table 5.4). Estimation of the TIBC can be helpful, since it is often below the normal range in the anaemia of chronic disease, and frequently above it in iron deficiency. If it is found to be within the normal range, then it does not provide help in the diagnosis. Serum ferritin levels are low in iron deficiency and normal or increased in chronic disorders. The degree of microcytosis is sometimes useful, since an MCV below 70 fl is much more likely to be due to iron deficiency than a chronic disorder.

The cause of the anaemia is not yet well-defined, but three factors have been established (Cartwright & Lee 1971):

1   A moderate decrease in the life-span of the red cells due to extracorpuscular factors.

2   An inadequate increase in erythropoietin production for the degree of anaemia leading to a suboptimal increase in erythropoietic activity.

3   Failure to release iron from macrophages for new red-cell production, leading to the formation of hypochromic microcytes.

4   An inhibition of erythroid progenitor cell proliferation by a serum factor or a product of bone marrow macrophages (in rheumatoid arthritis).

Sideroblastic anaemias

The term sideroblastic erythropoiesis is used to describe an abnormal type of red-cell production in which a substantial proportion of erythroblasts contain a perinuclear ring of coarse iron-containing granules (Fig. 5.7, Plate 11). These granules are not usually apparent in Romanowsky-stained marrow smears but appear blue in smears stained by Perls' acid ferrocyanide method for haemo-siderin. The abnormal cells are described as ringed sideroblasts. Ultrastructural studies have show that the granules within ringed sideroblasts consist of iron-laden mitochrondria; the iron-containing material is deposited in between the mitochondrial cristae (Fig. 5.8).

Sideroblastic erythropoiesis may be found both as an inherited (usually X-linked recessive) and an acquired condition. The abnormality occurs as an acquired condition in primary sideroblastic anaemia (also called refractory anaemia with ringed sideroblasts) (p. 110) and occasional patients with chronic myeloproliferative disorders or malignant disease. Acquired sideroblastic anaemia may also be secondary to excessive alcohol consumption, therapy with certain drugs (e.g. isoniazid or chloramphenicol), and lead poisoning. In some patients with hereditary sideroblastic anaemia, the MCV is markedly reduced and all the red cells show hypochromia and microcytosis. However, most patients with sideroblastic anaemia have a normal or increased MCV, only a small proportion of their red cells being hypochromic microcytes.

IRON OVERLOAD

As the body has no mechanism for actively increasing iron excretion, a progressive increase in total body iron stores occurs in two categories of patients:

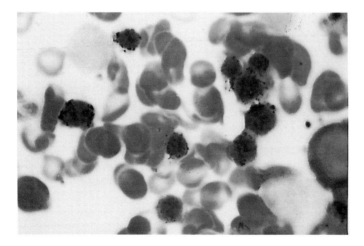

Fig. 5.7 Marrow smear from a patient with primary acquired sideroblastic anaemia, stained by Perls' acid ferrocyanide method (Prussian blue reaction). The erythroblasts contain several coarse (blue-black) iron-containing granules which are often arranged around the nucleus.

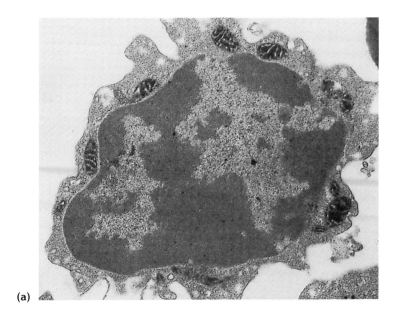

(a)

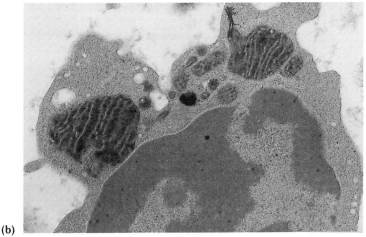

(b)

Fig. 5.8 Electron micrographs of two ringed sideroblasts from a patient with myelomatosis who developed sideroblastic erythropoiesis. (a) Perinuclear ring of iron-laden mitochondria. (b) Part of a ringed sideroblast photographed at higher magnification than (a), showing very electron-dense material between the cristae of enlarged mitochondria.

1   those who absorb increased quantities of iron over a prolonged period;
2   those receiving repeated blood transfusions over several years for conditions such as β-thalassaemia major, aplastic anaemia and pure red-cell aplasia. Iron absorption from a normal diet is inappropriately increased from birth in the condition known as idiopathic haemochromatosis in which there is an inherited error of iron metabolism. Affected patients usually develop symptoms between

the ages of 40 and 60 years. Iron absorption is also increased in patients with severe erythroid hyperplasia due to peripheral haemolysis or ineffectiveness of erythropoiesis. Some patients in the latter category (e.g. with thalassaemia intermedia or inherited sideroblastic anaemia) may have iron overload even when they have not been transfused to any significant extent.

When the iron stores become greatly increased (Plate 12), the heart, liver, endocrine organs and other tissues undergo progressive damage. Clinicopathological manifestations of severe iron overload include a bronze skin pigmentation, cardiac dysfunction, cirrhosis, diabetes mellitus, testicular atrophy and arthropathy.

The serum ferritin level is the most useful screening test for iron overload, being roughly proportional to the iron stores; it may be as high as 10 000 μg/l in severely affected patients. High serum ferritin levels may, however, be found in the presence of normal stores in conditions such as malignancy, infection and hepatocellular damage. The diagnosis of iron overload should be confirmed by liver biopsy which permits both the chemical estimation of the quantity of iron in the tissue and a histological assessment of the distribution of haemosiderin and the extent of tissue damage.

Idiopathic haemochromatosis is treated by repeated phlebotomy. Iron overload secondary to blood transfusion should be prevented or limited by the administration of the iron chelator desferrioxamine (p. 47). Patients who are developing iron overload secondary to increased erythropoietic activity should also be treated with desferrioxamine.

OBJECTIVES IN LEARNING

1   To know about the mechanisms of absorption, site of storage and method of plasma transportation of iron and the mechanism and extent of iron loss in men and women.

2   To know the causes of iron deficiency at all ages and in both sexes.

3   To know the mode of presentation of iron-deficiency anaemia.

4   To know the changes in the morphology of the red cells, in the red-cell indices, in the plasma iron levels and in the bone marrow associated with iron deficiency.

5   To know how to differentiate between the anaemia due to chronic disorders and that due to iron deficiency.

6   To know the principle of treatment of iron deficiency, both by the oral and parenteral routes.

7   To know the causes of hypochromic microcytic red cells other than iron deficiency.

8   To understand the causes and consequences of iron overload.

REFERENCES

Afifi A.M., Banwell G.S., Bennison R.J., Boothby K., Griffiths P.D., Huntsman R.G.(1966) Simple test for ingested iron in hospital and domiciliary practice. *Br. Med. J.*, **1**: 1021.

Aisen P. (1982) Current concepts in iron metabolism. *Clin. Haematol.*, **11**, 241.

Badenoch J., Callender, S.T. (1960) Effect of corticosteroids and gluten-free diet on absorption of iron in idiopathic steatorrhoea and coeliac disease. *Lancet*, i: 192.

Bainton D.F., Finch C.A. (1964) Diagnosis of iron deficiency. *Am. J. Med.*, **37**, 62.

Berry W.T.C., Nash F.A. (1954) Symptoms as a guide to anaemia. *Br. Med. J.*, **1**, 918.

Beutler E. (1959) Red cell indices in the diagnosis of iron deficiency anaemia. *Ann. Intern. Med.*, **50**, 313.

Beutler E., Robson M.J., Buttenweiser E. (1958) A comparison of plasma iron, iron-binding capacity, sternal marrow iron and other methods in the clinical evaluation of iron stores. *Ann. Intern. Med.*, **48**, 60.

Beveridge B.R., Bannerman R.M., Evanson J.M., Witts L.J. (1965) Hypochromic anaemia. *Q. J. Med.*, **34**, 145.

Brumfitt W. (1960) Primary iron-deficiency anaemia in young men. *Q. J. Med.*, **29**, 1.

Burman D. (1982) Iron deficiency in infants and childhood. *Clin. Haematol.*, **11**, 339.

Cartwright G.E., Lee G.R. (1971) The anaemia of chronic disorders. Annotation *Br. J. Haematol.*, **21**, 147.

Chanarin I., Rothman, D. (1965) Iron deficiency and its relation to folic-acid status in pregnancy: Results of a clinical trial. *Br. Med. J.*, **1**, 480.

Cook J.D., Alvarado J., Gutnisky A., Jamra M., Labardini J., Layrisse M. et al (1971) Nutritional deficiency and anaemia in Latin America. *Blood*, **38**, 591.

Cook J.D., Finch C.A., Smith N.J. (1976) Evaluation of the iron status of a population. *Blood*, **48**, 449.

Davis L.R., Marten R.H., Sarkany I. (1960) Iron-deficiency anaemia in European and West Indian infants in London. *Br. Med. J.*, **2**, 1426–8.

Elwood P.C., Jacobs A., Pitman R.G., Entwhistle C.C. (1964a) Epidemiology of the Paterson–Kelly syndrome. *Lancet*, ii: 716.

Elwood P.C., Withey J.L. Kilpatrick G.S. (1964b) Distribution of haemoglobin level in a group of schoolchildren and its relation to height, weight, and other variables. *Br. J. Prev. Soc. Med.*, **18**, 125.

Finch C.A., Loden, B. (1959) Body iron exchange in man. *J. Clin. Invest.* **38**, 392.

Foulkes J., Goldie D.J., (1982) The use of ferritin to assess the need for iron supplements in pregnancy. *J. Obstet. Gynaecol.*, **3**; 11–16.

Fry J. (1961) Clinical patterns and course of anaemia in general practice. *Br. Med. J.*, **2**, 1732.

Garby L., Ionell L., Werner I. (1969) Iron deficiency in women of fertile age in a Swedish community. *Acta Med. Scand.*, **185**, 113.

Giles C. & Burton H. (1960) Observation on prevention and diagnosis of anaemia in pregnancy. *Br. Med. J.*, **2**, 636.

Girdwood R.H. (1952) Treatment of anaemia. *Br. Med. J.*, **1**, 599.

Goldberg A., Lochhead A.C., Dagg J.H. (1963) Histamine-fast achlorhydria and iron absorption. *Lancet*, i, 848.

Halberg L., Hoogdaht A.M., Nilsson L., Rybo G. (1966) Menstrual blood loss and iron deficiency. *Acta Med. Scand.*, **180**, 639–50.

Hamilton L.D., Gubler C.J., Cartwright G.E., Wintrobe M.M. (1950) Diurnal variation in the plasma iron level of Man. *Proc. Soc. Exp. Biol. Med.*, **75**, 65.

Holt J.M., Gear M.W.L., Warner G.T. (1970) The role of chronic blood loss in the pathogenesis of postgastrectomy iron-deficiency anaemia. *Gut*, **11**, 847.

Jacobs A., Kilpatrick G.S. (1964) The Paterson–Kelly syndrome. *Br. Med. J.*, **2**, 79.

Jacobs A., Kilpatrick G.S. Withey J. L. (1965) Iron-deficiency anaemia in adults, prevalence and prevention. *Postgrad. Med. J.*, **41**, 418.

Jacobs A., Waters W.E., Campbell H. & Barrow A. (1969) A random sample from Wales. *Br. J. Haemaol.*, **17**, 581.

Newton M., Mosey L.M., Egii G.E., Gifford W.B., Hull C.T., (1961) Blood loss during and immediately after delivery. *Obstet. Gynecol.*, **17**, 9–18.

Scott D.E.I., Pritchard J.A. (1967) Iron deficiency in healthy college women. *J. Am. Med. Ass.*, **199**, 897.

Stevens A.R. (1958) In: *Iron in Clinical Medicine* (eds R.O. Wallerstein & S.R. Mettler). University of California Press.

Tovey F.I., Clark C.G. (1980) Anaemia after partial gastrectomy: a neglected curable condition. *Lancet* i: 956.

Verloop M.C., (1970) Iron depletion without anaemia: a controversial subject. *Blood* **36**; 657.

Walters G.O., Miller F.M., Worwood M. (1973) Serum ferritin concentrations and iron stores in normal subjects. *J. Clin. Pathol,* **26**, 770.

Zilva J.F. Patston V.J. (1966) Variation in serum-iron in healthy women. *Lancet*; **i**, 459–62.

Chapter 6
Macrocytosis and Macrocytic Anaemia

Macrocytosis and macrocytic anaemia may be found in a variety of unrelated diseases. In some conditions associated with macrocytosis, the red-cell precursors have a normal morphology (i.e. there is normoblastic erythropoiesis) and in others they show morphological abnormalities of the type seen in vitamin B_{12} deficiency associated with pernicious anaemia. Marrows containing such abnormal erythroblasts are described as displaying megaloblastic erythropoiesis. During the investigation of the cause of a macrocytic anaemia it is often helpful to determine the type of erythropoiesis by examining stained smears of bone marrow cells obtained by aspiration biopsy.

MEGALOBLASTIC ERYTHROPOIESIS

The causes of megaloblastic erythropoiesis are: (a) a deficiency of vitamin B_{12} or folate; (b) disturbances of vitamin B_{12} or folate metabolism; and (c) biochemical abnormalities unrelated to vitamin B_{12} or folate.

Megaloblastic erythropoiesis is characterized by abnormal red-cell precursors known as megaloblasts, in which cell and nuclear diameters are larger than those in normal red-cell precursors (normoblasts) and in which the condensed nuclear chromatin is more finely dispersed than in normoblasts of corresponding cytoplasmic maturity (Fig. 6.1, Plates 13, 14). Marrows showing megaloblastic erythropoiesis also frequently contain giant metamyelocytes. These are about twice the size of normal metamyelocytes and have horse-shoe-shaped or long,

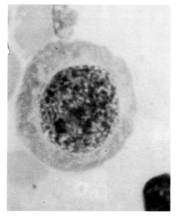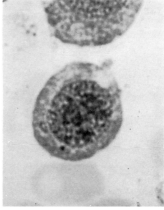

Fig. 6.1 Early polychromatic megaloblasts from a patient with severe pernicious anaemia. These cells are larger and have smaller granules of condensed nuclear chromatin than the two early polychromatic normoblasts in Fig. 1.2c on p. 4.

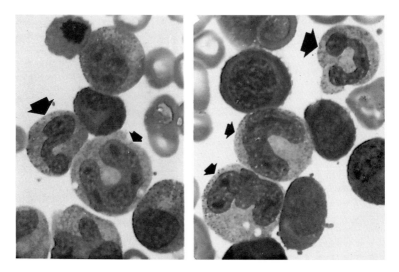

Fig. 6.2 Giant metamyelocytes (small arrows) near normal-sized metamyelocytes (large arrows) in a marrow smear from a patient with untreated pernicious anaemia. One of the giant metamyelocytes has an E-shaped nucleus.

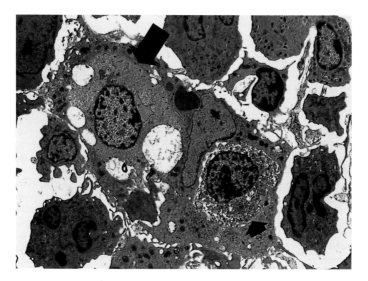

Fig. 6.3 Electron micrograph of a bone marrow macrophage from a patient with severe pernicious anaemia. The cytoplasm of the macrophage contains two ingested megaloblasts (arrowed) at various stages of degradation.

twisted, ribbon-like nuclei (Fig. 6.2). Morphological abnormalities may also be seen in megakaryocytes.

Megaloblasts suffer from a gross disturbance of cell proliferation and many of the more mature megaloblasts are ingested and degraded by bone marrow macrophages (Fig. 6.3). Thus, despite the fact that megaloblastic marrows show erythroid hyperplasia, this increased ineffectiveness of erythropoiesis (p. 5) results in the rate of delivery of new red cells into the circulation being suboptimal for the degree of anaemia. Many of the giant metamyelocytes are also destroyed within the marrow (ineffective granulocytopoiesis) (Wickramasinghe 1972).

Megaloblastic changes occur when DNA synthesis is disordered, but the detailed biochemical basis of the morphological abnormality remains uncertain. The ways in which vitamin B_{12} and folate deficiency may impair DNA synthesis are discussed later (p. 87 and p. 96).

In vitamin B_{12} and folate deficiency, megaloblastic changes are not confined to bone marrow cells; the characteristic nuclear abnormality is found in a variety of epithelial cells, including those of the buccal and nasal mucosa, tongue, urinary tract, jejunum, vagina and cervix uteri.

BLOOD PICTURE IN PATIENTS WITH MEGALOBLASTIC HAEMOPOIESIS

Some patients have a high MCV without anaemia. However, even in these patients the haemoglobin level may rise following the correction of the underlying defect indicating that their haemoglobin at presentation, although within the normal range, was below their own normal value. In other patients the high MCV is associated with varying degrees of anaemia. The absolute reticulocyte count is variable, being either reduced, normal or slightly increased. Any increase is much less than that seen in an individual with normally functioning bone marrow and a similar degree of anaemia. Red cell life-span is slightly decreased. The anaemia is mainly due to the ineffectiveness of megaloblastic erythropoiesis. The blood films of patients with megaloblastic erythropoiesis contain macrocytes, some of which are oval in shape (Fig. 6.4).

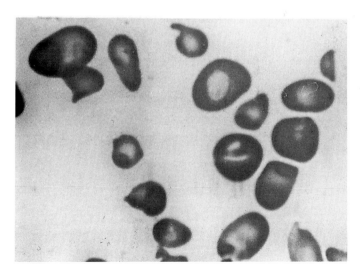

Fig. 6.4 Blood film from a patient with pernicious anaemia showing oval macrocytes and other poikilocytes

The red cells also show anisocytosis and poikilocytosis, particularly in moderately and severely anaemic cases. Macrocytic anaemias caused by megaloblastic haemopoiesis are referred to as megaloblastic anaemias.

In patients with vitamin B_{12}- or folate-related megaloblastic haemopoiesis, the circulating neutrophil granulocytes frequently show hypersegmentation of their nuclei (Fig. 6.5). Under normal circumstances, 3% or less of neutrophil granulocytes have five or more nuclear segments, but in vitamin B_{12} or folic-acid deficiency more than 3% are hypersegmented and there may even be occasional cells with eight or ten segments. Hypersegmentation is not diagnostic of vitamin B_{12} or folate deficiency; it may also occur in anaemia due to iron deficiency and in renal failure, even when B_{12} and folate stores are adequate. Hypersegmented neutrophil polymorphs are not derived from giant metamyelocytes but from normal-looking metamyelocytes. When the megaloblastic changes caused by vitamin B_{12} or folate deficiency are severe, there may be neutropenia and thrombocytopenia (due to ineffective granulocytopoiesis and thrombocytopoiesis).

MEGALOBLASTIC ANAEMIAS (MACROCYTIC ANAEMIAS WITH MEGALOBLASTIC ERYTHROPOIESIS)

Vitamin B_{12} deficiency

Biochemical and nutritional aspects of vitamin B_{12}

Biochemistry

The B_{12} molecule is composed of: (a) a planar corrin nucleus made up of four pyrrole rings (A–D); (b) the ribonucleotide of 5,6-dimethylbenzimidazole; and (c) a cobalt atom situated at the centre of the corrin nucleus which is coordinately bonded to the four pyrrole rings, one of the nitrogen atoms of the

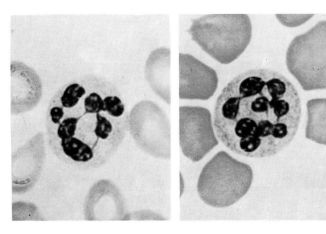

Fig. 6.5 Two hypersegmented neutrophil polymorphs from the peripheral blood smear of a patient with vitamin B_{12} deficiency due to pernicious anaemia.

ribonucleotide and to an organic group (Fig. 6.6). In the two biologically active forms of vitamin B_{12}, namely methylcobalamin and adenosylcobalamin, the organic groups bound to the cobalt atom are methyl and adenosyl, respectively.

The biochemical mechanisms underlying the clinical manifestations of vitamin B_{12} deficiency (anaemia, peripheral neuropathy and subacute combined degeneration of the spinal cord) are still uncertain. One of the two reactions known to require vitamin B_{12} in man is the methylation of homocysteine to methionine which is dependent both on 5-methyltetrahydrofolate and methylcobalamin. Since the 5-methyltetrahydrofolate serves as the methyl donor, failure of this reaction would result not only in impaired methionine synthesis but also in the accumulation of 5-methyltetrahydrofolate. It is generally held that impairment of this methyltransferase reaction in vitamin B_{12} deficiency eventually leads to a reduction in the availability of 5,10-methylenetetrahydrofolate for the conversion of deoxyuridylate to thymidylate, impaired DNA synthesis due to an inadequate supply of thymidylate triphosphate and, consequently, megaloblastic haemopoiesis. Nevertheless, there are also data indicating that impaired thymidylate synthesis may not be the critical defect underlying the megaloblastic change.

The mechanism by which an impairment of the homocysteine-methionine methyltransferase reaction may result in reduced levels of 5,10-methylene tetrahydrofolate was thought to be the trapping of intracellular folates in the form of 5-methyltetrahydrofolate which cannot be converted to 5,10-methylenetetrahydrofolate (methylfolate trap hypothesis). However, recent data have raised doubts regarding the validity of this hypothesis (Chanarin et al. 1980).

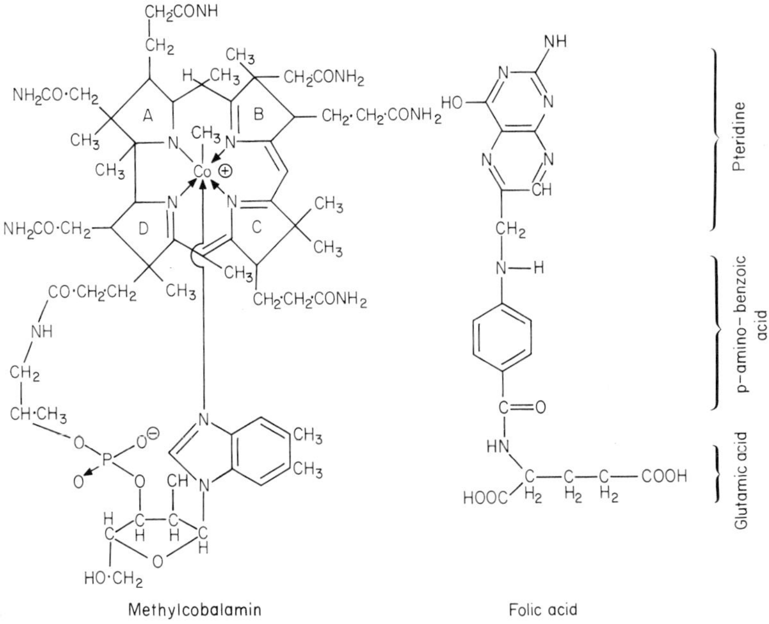

Fig. 6.6   The structure of vitamin B_{12} and folic acid.

Vitamin B_{12} in the diet

Vitamin B_{12} is produced entirely by bacteria and none is present in plants. Herbivora obtain vitamin B_{12} mainly as the result of synthesis by bacteria in their rumen; other animals and man obtain it by eating animal food. The average amount of B_{12} in a mixed diet is about 5 µg/day.

Mechanism of absorption

About 70% of 1µg of labelled native B_{12} in meat is absorbed. A decreasing proportion is absorbed as the quantity of B_{12} is increased; the maximum quantity that can be absorbed after a single meal is 2–3 µg.

Vitamin B_{12} ingested in physiological amounts is not absorbed unless it is first combined with intrinsic factor. The function of this factor is the transport of B_{12} into the epithelial cells of the distal half of the small intestine.

Intrinsic factor is produced in the body and fundus of the stomach by the same cells that produce hydrochloric acid, namely, the gastric parietal cells. Chemically, intrinsic factor is a glycoprotein with a molecular weight of about 44 000 and each molecule binds one molecule of B_{12}. The amount of intrinsic factor in the gastric juice can be estimated indirectly by measuring the amount of vitamin B_{12} that it can bind. The amount secreted in the absence of any stimulus each day is in the order of 70 000 units. The average basal secretion of 3000 units per hour increases 3–5-fold after the administration of stimulants such as histamine and gastrin. The quantity of vitamin B_{12} required to be absorbed daily to maintain body stores is about 1–3 µg, and only 1000–3000 units of intrinsic factor are necessary for its absorption. Thus, the amount of intrinsic factor produced daily is considerably in excess of that required for vitamin B_{12} absorption (Ardeman & Chanarin 1965). The minimum quantity of B_{12} that must be absorbed daily to maintain health (rather than to maintain body stores) may be less than 0.5 µg.

Storage and rate of loss of vitamin B_{12}

Vitamin B_{12} is mainly stored in the liver and the average healthy adult has a total body content of 3–5mg. Loss of vitamin B_{12} takes place in the urine and faeces mainly through desquamation of epithelial cells and through excretion in the bile.

The rate of loss of vitamin B_{12} is approximately 0.05–0.1% of the body content each day. There is therefore a delay of 2 years or more between the appearance of a lesion leading to impaired absorption of B_{12} and the reduction of the B_{12} store to a level (possibly about 300–500 µg) which causes megaloblastic anaemia. For instance, following the abrupt cessation of B_{12} as a consequence of total gastrectomy, it takes about 2–7 years before megaloblastic anaemia develops.

Vitamin B_{12} neuropathy

Patients with vitamin B_{12} deficiency due to the lack of gastric intrinsic factor or any other cause may develop degenerative changes in the nervous system (Pant *et al.* 1968). The pathological changes are often considered under three headings:

1 peripheral neuropathy;
2 subacute combined degeneration of the cord;
3 focal demyelinisation of the white matter of the brain.

In subacute combined degeneration of the cord there is patchy degeneration of the posterior and lateral columns which is most marked in (but not confined to) the lower cervical and upper thoracic segments (Fig. 6.7). The name subacute combined degeneration of the cord is, however, misleading since the onset of the symptoms is usually insidious and not subacute, lesions of the posterior and lateral columns can occur alone and are not necessarily combined, and the syndrome frequently includes lesions of the peripheral nerves or cerebral hemispheres as well as the spinal cord.

Symptoms and signs usually affect the lower limbs first and are symmetrical. The commonest symptoms are paraesthesiae and muscle weakness. Others include ataxia, stiffness of the limbs, impotence and impairment of bladder and rectal control. Some impairment of memory, irritability, mild depression, apathy and fluctuations of mood are relatively common but serious psychiatric symptoms (e.g. stupor, hallucinations, paranoia, severe depression and manic psychosis) are uncommon. However, some patients have been rescued from mental institutions and restored to health by B_{12} injections.

On the basis of a clinical examination of the nervous system, it is sometimes difficult to distinguish with certainty between peripheral neuritis and posterior column involvement, since in both conditions tendon reflexes and vibrational and positional sense may be reduced, and ataxia may be present. However, hyperalgesia of calf muscles favours peripheral neuritis, whereas a disproportionate reduction in positional and vibrational sense up to the pelvis compared

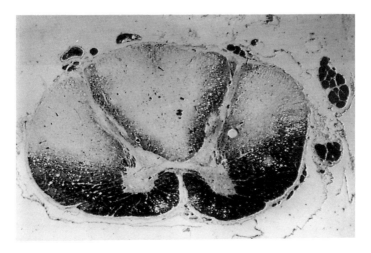

Fig. 6.7 Subacute combined degeneration of the cervical spinal cord. The posterior and lateral columns show demyelination and, therefore, appear pale (Weigert–Pal method for myelin). (With permission from Dr RO Barnard.)

to touch and pin-prick favours involvement of the lateral columns. An extensor plantar response indicates pyramidal tract involvement. Individual patients varyas to the extent to which lesions in the posterior columns, lateral columns, or peripheral nerves dominate the neurological syndrome. Spinal cord lesions may predominate in the absence of peripheral neuritis and vice versa. Optic atrophy has been reported but is rare.

Neurological involvement may occur without anaemia although the bone marrow usually shows mild megaloblastic changes.

Causes of vitamin B_{12} deficiency

These are summarized in Table 6.1. The two most common mechanisms of vitamin B_{12} deficiency are a failure to secrete intrinsic factor and a failure to absorb vitamin B_{12} as a result of abnormalities in the distal ileum.

Inadequate intake

Veganism

Vitamin B_{12} deficiency resulting from a very low B_{12} content in the diet only occurs in strict vegetarians who eat no animal protein at all (vegans). Although there is no vitamin B_{12} in plants, the vegan diet probably contains some B_{12} as a result of bacterial contamination of water and vegetables and bacterial fermentation of bruised vegetables. Low serum vitamin B_{12} levels are found in over 50% of vegans. However, most vegans with low serum B_{12} levels are healthy and do not show anaemia or macrocytosis; only a minority suffer from megaloblastic anaemia or vitamin B_{12} neuropathy.

Table 6.1.   Mechanisms and causes of vitamin B_{12} deficiency.

Inadequate intake
Veganism

Inadequate secretion of intrinsic factor
Pernicious anaemia
Total or partial gastrectomy
Congenital intrinsic factor deficiency (rare)

Diversion of dietary B_{12}
Abnormal intestinal bacterial flora
    multiple jejunal diverticula, small intestinal
    strictures, stagnant intestinal loops
Diphyllobothrium latum

Malabsorption
Crohn's disease, ileal resection,
    chronic tropical sprue, congenital
    selective B_{12} malabsorption with
    proteinuria (Imerslund–Gräsbeck syndrome)

Inadequate secretion of intrinsic factor

Pernicious anaemia

Aetiology and pathogenesis

Pernicious anaemia is a condition in which the absorption of vitamin B_{12} is markedly reduced due to a failure or severe reduction of intrinsic factor secretion secondary to severe atrophic gastritis or gastric atrophy. The basal secretion of intrinsic factor is reduced to only 0–200 units per hour and is unaffected by stimulants such as histamine. Vitamin B_{12} deficiency develops and leads to megaloblastic anaemia, neurological damage, or both. The disease was first described by Thomas Addison of Guy's Hospital, London, in 1849, and is therefore sometimes referred to as Addisonian pernicious anaemia. About 20% of patients have a relative with pernicious anaemia, suggesting that genetic factors play an important role in the development of this disease. Individuals with the genetic defect may have an inborn susceptibility to develop gastric atrophy in adult life. Antibodies against gastric parietal cells are found in the serum in about 85% of patients with pernicious anaemia. Furthermore, antibodies against intrinsic factor are found in the serum of about 55% of patients and in the gastric juice of about 60%. However, the fact that such antibodies cannot be detected in all cases, combined with the observation that a few patients with thyroid disorders have anti-intrinsic factor antibodies in their serum but do not have B_{12} deficiency, suggest that these antibodies are not the primary cause of the gastric atrophy and the resulting failure of intrinsic factor secretion; they may instead be a consequence of the damage to the gastric mucosa. It is possible on the other hand that the gastric atrophy is the result of cell-mediated immune reactions against parietal and other gastric cells.

All cases of pernicious anaemia have a gastric lesion, varying from severe atrophic gastritis to gastric atrophy. As both intrinsic factor and hydrochloric acid are produced by the same cell (i.e. the parietal cell), it is not surprising that histamine-fast and pentagastrin-fast achlorhydria is an invariable accompaniment of pernicious anaemia and the diagnosis cannot be made if appreciable quantities of hydrochloric acid are found to be secreted. The pH of resting gastric juice in pernicious anaemia is between 6 and 8 and after maximal stimulation with histamine or pentagastrin it does not fall by more than 0.5 pH units. However, not all individuals with gastric atrophy or achlorhydria have pernicious anaemia, presumably because many individuals with these abnormalities continue to secrete the small quantities of intrinsic factor required for the absorption of adequate amounts of B_{12}.

Pernicious anaemia should not be regarded merely as a condition in which there is a deficient production of red cells and damage to the nervous system but rather as a vitamin deficiency disease affecting many cell types in the body, including all dividing cells. Symptoms and signs are referable not only to the blood and neural tissue (brain, spinal cord, peripheral nerves), but also to the gastrointestinal tract (from the tongue down to the colon), skin and other tissues and organs (e.g. ovaries). Severe anaemia may aggravate co-existing cardiac disease.

Clinical features

Pernicious anaemia is most common in people of Northern European extraction and in England its prevalence is about 1 per 1000 of the population. Only 10% of cases are diagnosed under 40 years of age; the prevalence increases with age, reaching around 1% between the ages of 70 and 79 years. Females are 1.5 times more frequently affected than males.

Symptoms develop slowly. Davidson (1957) found the four most common presenting symptoms were tiredness and weakness (90% of patients), dyspnoea (70%), paraesthesia (38%) and sore tongue (25%). Although many patients complained of vague gastrointestinal disturbance (anorexia, nausea, vomiting, dyspepsia, constipation), diarrhoea only occurred in 9%. Loss of weight is seen in some cases (Seaton & Goldberg 1960). Other symptoms include subfertility and, rarely, hyperpigmentation of the skin of the hands. Apart from pallor, the most frequent sign was atrophic glossitis (64%). Commonly, some degree of papillary atrophy of the tongue is seen as an unusual smoothness at the edges, but this sometimes spreads over the entire dorsal surface (Fig. 6.8). Occasionally, the tongue is red, painful and ulcerated. Fever was present in 22% and the spleen was slightly enlarged in 8% of the cases; usually only the tip was felt. Various neurological and psychiatric symptoms may develop in a small proportion of cases, due to a vitamin B_{12} neuropathy (p. 89). Male patients with pernicious anaemia have an increased incidence of gastric carcinoma.

Haematological and biochemical changes

The blood picture is that seen in any vitamin B_{12}- or folate-related megaloblastic anaemia (p. 85). The haemoglobin level may be within the normal range in patients diagnosed early but decreases progressively as the degree of deficiency increases. The blood count shows a high MCV provided that the pernicious anaemia is not complicated by co-existing conditions such as iron deficiency or

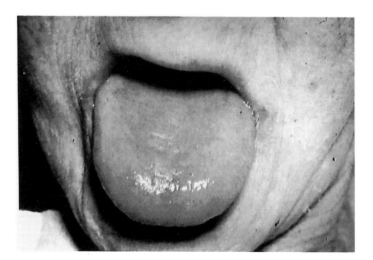

Fig. 6.8   Glossitis in a woman with severe pernicious anaemia.

thalassaemia trait. The marrow is hypercellular and in severely anaemic patients virtually all of the fat cells of the marrow are replaced by haemopoietic cells. Haemopoiesis is megaloblastic in type (p. 83) and giant metamyelocytes may be present. In marrow smears stained by Perls' acid ferrocyanide method, the quantity of haemosiderin within the marrow fragments is usually either normal or increased.

There may be a slight increase in the serum bilirubin level and an increase in serum lactate dehydrogenase; these changes result mainly from the intramedullary destruction of erythroblasts and partly from a mild degree of peripheral haemolysis. The level of B_{12} in the serum is virtually always reduced. However, low serum B_{12} levels should be considered as presumptive rather than definitive evidence of B_{12} deficiency, since they are also found in the absence of any other evidence of B_{12} deficiency, in one-third of folate-deficient patients and in some pregnant women and elderly individuals. About 60% of patients with pernicious anaemia have low red cell folate levels and the remainder have normal levels.

Diagnosis (see Table 6.2 on p. 96)

Pernicious anaemia cannot be reliably diagnosed on the patient's history and clinical examination alone. Davidson (1957) concluded that 'there are no pathognomonic symptoms or signs which will establish the diagnosis of pernicious anaemia; that tiredness, breathlessness, paraesthesia and chronic atrophic glossitis are presenting features which occur frequently in other types of anaemia and in particular in some cases of iron-deficiency anaemia'. In order to establish the diagnosis of pernicious anaemia with certainty, it is necessary to demonstrate either a marked reduction or the absence of intrinsic factor in gastric juice. This is usually done indirectly by performing a Schilling test (Schilling 1953). This test measures the ability of an individual to absorb orally administered cyanocobalamin. It involves giving 1 µg of ^{57}Co-cyanocobalamin by mouth and, at the same time, 1000 µg of non-radioactive cyanocobalamin intramuscularly. The urine passed over the next 24 hours is collected and its radioactivity determined. The large intramuscular dose of non-radioactive B_{12} saturates the B_{12}-binding proteins in the plasma and thus causes a substantial proportion of any absorbed ^{57}Co-B_{12} to be excreted in the urine. B_{12} absorption is considered to be impaired when the urinary excretion of ^{57}Co-B_{12} over the 24 hours is less than 10% of the dose given by mouth. In pernicious anaemia it is often below 5%. If the test is abnormal it should be repeated giving both intrinsic factor and ^{57}Co-B_{12} by mouth; if the low B_{12} absorption in the patient is the result of intrinsic factor deficiency, then the absorption will be improved (but not restored to normal). This test clearly gives essential information concerning the basic defect in pernicious anaemia and is the most important of all the tests that can be performed. The diagnosis of pernicious anaemia can be more directly established by assay of intrinsic factor secretion in gastric juice but this procedure has been replaced by the simpler Schilling test and is no longer in routine use.

Treatment

Patients with pernicious anaemia should be initially treated with 1000 µg hydroxocobalamin intramuscularly every 2–3 weeks over a period of 2–3 months. Maintenance therapy with injections of 1000 μg hydroxocobalamin every 2 months should be continued for the rest of their lives. It is customary to start treating patients with serious neurological symptoms with 1000 μg hydroxocobalamin twice a week rather than every 2–3 weeks. The use of cyanocobalamin in the treatment of pernicious anaemia has now been discontinued since plasma levels of vitamin B_{12} are maintained for longer periods after the injection of a given dose of hydroxocobalamin when compared with the same dose of cyanocobalamin (Tudhope et al. 1967). Complicating infections and congestive cardiac failure should be treated promptly. Blood transfusion should be avoided whenever possible as this may precipitate or aggravate cardiac failure. If transfusion is necessary in severely anaemic patients, this should be done cautiously under cover of diuretics, administering no more than 1–2 units of packed red cells slowly over 24 hours. Some clinicians prefer to perform a 1–2 unit partial exchange transfusion. A number of patients with severe pernicious anaemia die suddenly, presumably of cardiac arrhythmias, shortly after the start of B_{12} therapy and this has been attributed to a fall in serum potassium consequent on a movement of potassium into cells in response to therapy with B_{12}. Patients with severe pernicious anaemia should therefore be started on oral potassium supplements at the same time as the B_{12}; the potassium should be continued for 10 days. If the cause of a severe megaloblastic anaemia is uncertain at presentation, as is often the case, treatment should be started with both hydroxocobalamin intramuscularly and folic acid orally. It must be emphasized that B_{12} deficiency should not be treated for a prolonged period with folic acid alone since, although the anaemia usually responds, neurological lesions do not and may rapidly progress.

Response to hydroxocobalamin is rapid. There is an increase in mental acuity and a sense of well-being within 24–48 hours. The reticulocyte response peaks at about 5–7 days (Fig. 6.9) and, after the first week, the haemoglobin rises by about 1 g/week. Neurological symptoms of recent onset (less than about 3 months duration) show marked improvement and may even disappear over the

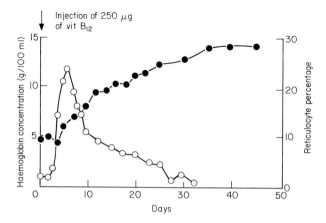

Fig. 6.9 Response of a patient with pernicious anaemia to vitamin B_{12} administration: (●), haemoglobin concentration; (○), reticulocyte percentage.

first 6–12 months of therapy. More long-standing symptoms improve to a lesser extent. Mental symptoms often disappear rapidly and completely.

Total or partial gastrectomy

Megaloblastic anaemia due to vitamin B_{12} deficiency is an invariable result of total gastrectomy and develops 2–10 years after the operation, this being the time taken to exhaust the B_{12} stores present preoperatively. Deficiency may also develop after partial gastrectomy but usually not before 5 years have elapsed, and is due to the removal of most of the intrinsic factor-producing area of the stomach and atrophy of the remaining mucosa. The incidence of deficiency after partial gastrectomy is sufficiently high to warrant routine periodic examination of the blood in all patients. Deller & Witts (1962) investigated 285 patients with partial gastrectomy for up to 12 years following the operation and found 54 who were anaemic. In most of the patients the anaemia was due to iron deficiency, but 5% of all the patients examined had evidence of B_{12} deficiency and 2 of the patients had subacute combined degeneration of the cord.

Diversion of dietary B_{12}

Abnormal intestinal bacterial flora ('stagnant loop syndrome')

Macrocytic anaemia often arises in patients who have anatomical abnormalities of the small gut (blind loops, fistulae, diverticulosis, anastomoses and others) which lead to stasis and bacterial overgrowth. Many strains of bacteria found in stagnant small intestinal loops can take up B_{12} and convert it to inactive cobamides, leaving none for absorption by the host. Folic acid is not affected in this way: in fact folic acid may be produced by these bacteria and, therefore, red cell folate levels may be high. Patients with this condition give an abnormal result with the Schilling test for B_{12} absorption (both without and with intrinsic factor); the abnormality is corrected after therapy with broad-spectrum antibiotics.

Infestation with the fish tapeworm

Diversion of B_{12} in the gut can occur due to successful competition by the fish tape-worm, *Diphyllobothrium latum*, which was common in Finland, but is now becoming rare.

Malabsorption

Malabsorption of B_{12} due to disease of the terminal ileum may be seen in coeliac disease and regional ileitis, and is almost invariable in chronic tropical sprue. In the latter, B_{12} deficiency is often combined with folate deficiency. Reduced absorption of B_{12} also occurs after resection of the terminal ileum.

Diagnosis of vitamin B_{12} deficiency

The investigations that may be of diagnostic value in a patient suspected of suffering from vitamin B_{12} deficiency are given in Table 6.2; some of these are discussed in more detail in the preceding sections.

Table 6.2 Tests useful in establishing the diagnosis and cause of vitamin B_{12} deficiency.

Investigation	Findings
Blood count	High MCV
Blood film	Oval macrocytes, hypersegmentation of neutrophil granulocytes
Bone marrow aspiration	Megaloblasts, giant metamyelocytes
Serum vitamin B_{12}	Low
Red cell folate	Normal or low
Dietary assessment	No intake of animal protein in Vegans
Schilling test for B_{12} absorption	Abnormal in pernicious anaemia, diseases of the terminal ileum and in the 'stagnant loop syndrome'
Barium meal and follow through	Demonstrates various lesions of the small intestine in the 'stagnant loop syndrome' and in diseases of the terminal ileum
Assay of intrinsic factor in gastric juice	Very low or absent in pernicious anaemia.

Folate deficiency

Biochemical and nutritional aspects of folate

Biochemistry

Folic acid (pteroylmonoglutamic acid) is composed of three portions, a pteridine nucleus, p-aminobenzoic acid and glutamic acid (see Fig. 6.6). This compound is not biochemically active until it is reduced first to dihydrofolic acid and then to tetrahydrofolic acid. In addition, naturally occurring forms of folate contain a single carbon unit in various states of reduction (e.g. methyl, formyl, methylene). Whereas the folate present in the serum is 5-methyltetrahydrofolate monoglutamate, intracellular folates are pteroylpolyglutamates with 3–7 glutamic acid residues joined together. The active forms of folate function as coenzymes in the transfer of single carbon units in (a) amino acid metabolism; and (b) the synthesis of purines and pyrimidines required for DNA and RNA synthesis. In particular, 5,10-methylenetetrahydrofolate is required for the methylation of deoxyuridylate to thymidylate and an impairment of this reaction may be one of the biochemical abnormalities underlying the altered DNA synthesis and the megaloblastic change in folate deficiency (also see p. 87).

Folates in the diet

Folates are found in both animal and plant foods. An average Western diet contains daily about 400 µg of folate. The folate content of food is markedly affected by cooking as folates are rapidly destroyed by heat. About 80% of an oral dose of 200 µg pteroylglutamic acid is absorbed; the percentage absorption of polyglutamates is somewhat lower. In an adult, the minimum quantity of folate required to be absorbed daily is about 100–200 µg. The requirement is greater during pregnancy and lactation.

Absorption

This takes place mainly in the duodenum and jejunum. The folate polyglutamates in the diet are converted to monoglutamates by the action of the enzyme folate conjugase and the monoglutamates are converted to 5-methyltetrahydrofolate monoglutamate by the enterocyte before it reaches the portal blood stream.

Storage and rate of loss of folates

The hepatic store of folate is normally greater than that of vitamin B_{12}, being about 8–20 mg. Folate is lost from the body in cells shed from the skin and intestinal epithelium, and in bile, urine, sweat and saliva. Folate is also lost by intracellular catabolism. The rate of loss of folate is approximately 1–2% of the total hepatic stores per day, a rate which is 10–20 times greater than the rate of loss of B_{12}. Since the minimum amount of folate required to be absorbed per day is about 100 times greater than that of B_{12} and because folate turns over more rapidly than B_{12}, signs of folate deficiency appear much more rapidly than those of B_{12} deficiency. Thus, Herbert (1964) found that mildly megaloblastic haemopoiesis developed 5 months after a normal person was put on a folate-deficient diet, whereas it is known that after total gastrectomy, anaemia due to B_{12} deficiency does not develop for 2 years or more.

Factors causing folate deficiency

These are summarized in Table 6.3.

Inadequate diet

Megaloblastic anaemia due to inadequate intake of folate is seen in the poor, the elderly, the mentally disturbed, chronic alcoholics and infants fed on goats milk which is low in folate (goats milk anaemia).

Malabsorption

Since folate is absorbed in the upper part of the small intestine, diseases which affect this part such as coeliac disease and tropical sprue may cause megalo-

Table 6.3. Causes of folate deficiency.

Inadequate dietary intake

Malabsorption
  Coeliac disease, jejunal resection, tropical sprue

Increased requirement
  Pregnancy, premature infants, chronic haemolytic
  anaemias, myelofibrosis, various malignant diseases

blastic anaemia due to folate deficiency. Jejunal resection may also be followed by folate deficiency. In these malabsorption syndromes, folate deficiency is commonly associated with iron deficiency. This is because iron is absorbed by the same region of the small bowel as folate.

Increased requirement

Folate deficiency and megaloblastic anaemia are found whenever there is an increased demand for folate which is not met by absorption from an adequate diet. The increased requirement for folate may result from increased nucleic acid synthesis (e.g. pregnancy and chronic haemolytic anaemia) or from increased loss of folate from the body (e.g. infection with sustained pyrexia, desquamating skin diseases such as psoriasis).

Megaloblastic anaemia of pregnancy

Before the use of folate supplements during pregnancy, macrocytic anaemia due to folate deficiency was found in 0.5–5% of all pregnancies in the UK. However, examination of the bone marrow during pregnancy revealed that megaloblastic haemopoiesis was even more common, being found in about one-third of cases. The diagnosis of megaloblastic anaemia is usually made after the 36th week of gestation or during the first 4 weeks of the postpartum period. The prevalence of megaloblastic anaemia of pregnancy is much higher in developing countries than in the UK.

The chief cause of folate deficiency in pregnancy is the greatly increased DNA and RNA synthesis associated with the growth of the fetus, placenta and uterus, and the expansion of the red-cell mass of the mother. It has been calculated that folate requirements increase approximately three times during pregnancy (Editorial 1968). Several subsidiary factors also play a part. Giles (1966) found that about one-third of the patients had anorexia and thus presumably a reduced food intake. There also appears to be a reduction in folate absorption during pregnancy, and an increase in folate requirements may result from urinary infection.

Diagnosis of folate deficiency

The haematological features of folate deficiency are macrocytosis with or without anaemia, hypersegmentation of circulating neutrophil granulocytes and megaloblastic haemopoiesis (pp. 83–86). In order to establish that these changes are caused by folate deficiency rather than by any of the other causes of megaloblastic haemopoiesis, it is necessary to establish that the patient has reduced folate stores. This is usually done by measuring red cell folate levels. Serum folate levels are much less reliable than red cell folate levels in assessing folate stores as they are readily affected by a short period of negative folate balance. However, even a low red cell folate level cannot on its own be considered proof of folate deficiency since low values are found in 60% of vitamin B_{12}-deficient patients. In practice, therefore, the diagnosis of folate deficiency requires not only the finding of a low red cell folate level in the appropriate clinical setting but also the exclusion of vitamin B_{12} deficiency by demonstrating a normal serum B_{12} level or a normal Schilling test in those patients (other than pregnant women) with borderline or low serum vitamin B_{12} levels.

The diagnosis is confirmed by showing that the patient responds to treatment with folate. The cause of the folate deficiency is determined by taking a detailed dietary history and by performing tests of small intestinal function (including jejunal biopsy) when appropriate.

Treatment of folate deficiency

In an adult, macrocytosis or megaloblastic anaemia due to folate deficiency should be treated with 5 mg folic acid daily by mouth. The duration of treatment depends on the underlying disease but should, in any case, be at least 3 months. The initial haematological response is a reticulocytosis which peaks on the fifth to seventh day. The haemoglobin concentration must be followed until it reaches the normal range, because a few patients, especially those with the malabsorption syndrome, may also be vitamin B_{12}- or iron-deficient, and this can be detected by an incomplete rise in the haemoglobin level. Such patients show a second response when vitamin B_{12} or iron is added to their treatment.

DISTURBANCES IN VITAMIN B_{12} OR FOLATE METABOLISM

Nitrous oxide (N_2O) disturbs vitamin B_{12} metabolism by oxidising and inactivating methylcobalamin (Chanarin 1982). Continuous exposure of patients to a mixture of 50% N_2O and 50% O_2 for 5–24 hours often induces mild megaloblastic changes in the marrow. Intermittent exposure to N_2O for prolonged periods has caused a neuropathy in dentists working with, or addicted to, this gas. Drugs which inhibit dihydrofolate reductase (e.g. methotrexate and pyrimethamine) cause macrocytosis and megaloblastic changes by interfering with the regeneration of 5,10-methylenetetrahydrofolate from dihydrofolate. Megaloblastic haemopoiesis is also seen in some rare congenital disorders of vitamin B_{12} and folate metabolism.

VITAMIN B_{12}-INDEPENDENT AND FOLATE-INDEPENDENT CAUSES OF MEGALOBLASTIC HAEMOPOIESIS

A list of conditions causing megaloblastic haemopoiesis by mechanisms unrelated to vitamin B_{12} or folate is given in Table 6.4. The drugs listed interfere with nucleic acid synthesis. Orotic aciduria is a rare inherited disorder in which megaloblastic anaemia develops because of a reduced activity of enzymes involved in the conversion of orotic acid to uridine monophosphate. This leads to an impairment in the supply of pyrimidine bases for incorporation into DNA and RNA.

MACROCYTOSIS ASSOCIATED WITH NORMOBLASTIC ERYTHROPOIESIS

There are a number of conditions in which high MCVs may be associated with normoblastic erythropoiesis (Table 6.5). The most common of these, and indeed the commonest cause of macrocytosis in the UK, is chronic alcoholism.

Table 6.4.   Vitamin B_{12}-independent and folate-independent causes of macrocytosis with megaloblastic haemopoiesis.

Abnormalities of nucleic acid synthesis
Drug therapy
    Antipurines (mercaptopurine, azathioprine)
    Antipyrimidines (fluorouracil)
    Others (hydroxyurea, cyclophosphamide)
Orotic aciduria

Uncertain aetiology
Myelodysplastic syndromes, erythroleukaemia
Some congenital dyserythropoietic anaemias.

Table 6.5.   Causes of macrocytosis with normoblastic erythropoiesis.

Normal neonates (physiological)
Chronic alcoholism*
Chronic liver disease*
Haemolytic anaemia*
Hypothyroidism*
Therapy with anticonvulsant drugs*
Normal pregnancy
Chronic lung disease (with hypoxia)
Primary acquired sideroblastic anaemia*
Hypoplastic and aplastic anaemia

---

*Some patients show megaloblastic erythropoiesis

Chronic alcoholism

With the advent of automated blood counting machines which estimate red-cell indices on every blood sample analysed, relatively accurate estimates of MCV have become available on a large number of patients. Such data have revealed that the prevalence of macrocytosis not due to B_{12} or folate deficiency is higher than previously thought and that most individuals showing this abnormality consumed excess quantities of alcohol (Unger & Johnson 1974; Davidson & Hamilton 1978). It seems that the level of alcohol consumption that induces macrocytosis varies considerably in different individuals. Some individuals who consume about one-third of a bottle of spirits or its equivalent (80 g alcohol) each day develop high MCVs whereas others who consume as much as one bottle of spirits per day may not. Although some chronic alcoholics suffer from folate deficiency due to inadequate intake, the majority have neither B_{12} or folate deficiency, nor anaemia. When folate stores are adequate, erythropoiesis is usually normoblastic, not megaloblastic. It has been suggested that the macrocytosis is due to a toxic effect of acetaldehyde on erythroblasts. The acetaldehyde is probably generated locally by oxidation of ethanol by bone marrow macrophages. MCV values return to normal 2–3 months after stopping the high alcohol intake.

Haemolytic anaemia

Some patients with haemolytic anaemia develop increasing macrocytosis and megaloblastic haemopoiesis due to folate deficiency (p. 98). Other patients develop macrocytosis by a mechanism that is unrelated to folate deficiency. In the latter, the macrocytosis is associated with normoblastic erythropoiesis and is a manifestation of greatly accelerated erythropoiesis. The reticulocytes produced under these circumstances are larger than normal and mature into macrocytes which differ from those seen in vitamin B_{12} or folate deficiency in having rounded rather than oval outlines.

Hypothyroidism

There is a high frequency of thyroid and parietal cell antibodies in both hypothyroidism and pernicious anaemia and about 10% of all patients with hypothyroidism have pernicious anaemia. Patients with hypothyroidism may also develop macrocytosis by a mechanism which is based not on B_{12} or folate deficiency but on the deficiency of thyroxine. About one-quarter of patients with hypothyroidism (without associated pernicious anaemia) have an MCV above the normal range. Following the administration of thyroxine, all patients including those whose MCV is within the normal range, show a fall in MCV (Horton *et al.* 1976).

Anticonvulsant drugs

A high MCV is seen in some patients receiving phenytoin sodium (with or without other anticonvulsant drugs) and this may be associated either with megaloblastic or normoblastic erythropoiesis. In a proportion of patients with megaloblastic changes, the macrocytosis is caused by folate deficiency and such patients are often anaemic. In the other patients with megaloblastic changes and in all patients with normoblastic erythropoiesis, the macrocytosis is caused by an unknown mechanism independent of vitamin B_{12} and folate abnormalities; such patients are usually not anaemic.

OBJECTIVES IN LEARNING

1 To understand the relationship between the terms macrocytic, megaloblastic, B_{12} deficiency and folate deficiency.

2 To know the mechanisms of absorption, extent and site of storage, and the mechanism and rate of loss from the body of both B_{12} and folate.

3 To compare and contrast the causes of B_{12} deficiency with those of folate deficiency.

4 To know the symptoms and signs of pernicious anaemia referable to the gastrointestinal tract, central nervous system, peripheral nerves, and the cardiovascular and haematological systems.

5 To understand the principles involved in making the diagnosis of pernicious anaemia from various laboratory investigations.

6 To understand the method of differentiation of megaloblastic anaemia due to B_{12} deficiency from that due to folate deficiency.

7 To understand the principles of treatment with both B_{12} and folate.

8 To know the vitamin B_{12}- and folate-independent causes of macrocytosis.

REFERENCES

Ardeman S., Chanarin I. (1965) Assay of gastric intrinsic factor in the diagnosis of Addisonian pernicious anaemia. *Br. J. Haematol*, **11**: 306.

Chanarin I. (1982) The effects of nitrous oxide on cobalamins, folates and on related events. In: *CRC Critical Reviews on Toxicology*, pp. 179–213. CRC Press, Florida.

Chanarin I, Deacon R, Lumb M., Perry J. (1980) Vitamin B_{12} regulates folate metabolism by the supply of formate. *Lancet*, **2**: 505.

Chanarin I., Rothman D., Ward A., Perry J. (1968) Folate status and requirement in pregnancy. *Br. Med. J.*, **2**: 390.

Davidson R.J.L., Hamilton P.J. (1978) High mean cell volume, its incidence and significance in routine haematology. *J. Clin. Pathol.*, **31**: 395.

Davidson S. (1957) Clinical picture of pernicious anaemia prior to introduction of liver therapy in 1926 and in Edinburgh subsequent to 1944. *Br. Med. J.*, **1**: 241.

Deller L.J., Witts L.J. (1962) Changes in the blood after partial gastrectomy with special reference to vitamin B_{12}. *Q. J. Med.*, **31**: 71.

Editorial (1968) Nutritional folate deficiency. *Br. Med. J.*, **2**: 377.

Giles C. (1966) An account of 335 cases of megaloblastic anaemia of pregnancy and puerperium. *J. Clin. Pathol.*, **19**: 1.

Herbert V. (1964) Studies of folate deficiency in man. *Proc. R. Soc. Med.*, **57**: 377.

Horton L., Coburn R.J., England J.M., Himsworth R.L. (1976) The haematology of hypothyroidism. *Q. J. Med.*, **45**: 101.

Pant S.H., Ashbury A.K., Richardson E.P. (1968) The myelopathy of pernicious anaemia. A neuropathological reappraisal. *Acta Neurol. Scand.*, **44**, Suppl. 35, 1–36.

Schilling R.F. (1953) A new test for intrinsic factor activity. *J. Lab. Clin. Med.*, **42**: 946.

Seaton D.A., Goldberg A. (1960) Weight-loss in pernicious anaemia. *Lancet*, **i**, 002.

Tudhope G.R., Swan H.T., Spray G.H. (1967) Patient variation in pernicious anaemia as shown in a clinical trial of cyanocobalamin, hydroxycobalamin and cyanocobalamin-zinc-tannate. *Br. J. Haematol.*, **13**: 216.

Unger K.W., Johnson D., Jr. (1974) Red blood cell mean corpuscular volume: a potential indicator of alcohol usage in a working population. *Am. J. Med. Sci.*, **267**: 281.

Wickramasinghe S.N. (1972) Kinetics and morphology of haemopoiesis in pernicious anaemia (Annotation). *Br. J. Haematol.*, **22**: 111.

RECOMMENDED READING

Carmel R. (1983) Megaloblastic anaemia: vitamin B_{12} and folate. In: *Current Hematology* (ed. V.F. Fairbanks) vol. 2, pp. 243–80. John Wiley, New York.

Chanarin I. (1970) Pernicious anaemia and other vitamin B_{12} deficiency states. *Abst. of World Med.*, **44**: 73.

Chanarin I. (1979) *The Megaloblastic Anaemias* (2nd edn). Blackwell Scientific Publications, Oxford.

Editorial (1970) Management of megaloblastic anaemia. *Lancet*, **ii**: 27.

Chapter 7
Abnormalities of White Cells

In many pathological states, circulating white blood cells may show alterations in their morphology, function or concentration. Although changes in the absolute count of various types of white cell are commonly found in disease, and are usually non-specific, they may provide invaluable diagnostic clues. Alterations in white cells are most frequently associated with non-neoplastic disorders but may also be seen in the myelodysplastic syndromes (a pre-leukaemic state), in the chronic myeloproliferative disorders, and in various malignant diseases, including leukaemias.

LEUCOPENIA

The terms leucopenia and neutropenia are used to describe a reduction in the total white cell count and neutrophil count, respectively, to values below their normal ranges. The terms lymphocytopenia or lymphopenia are used when the lymphocyte count is subnormal.

Neutropenia

Selective neutropenia may occur in a large number of conditions (Table 7.1). In particular, it may be found in patients receiving various drugs, many of which are in common use. There is a substantial risk of serious infection when the neutrophil count falls below 0.5×10^9/litre.

Neutropenia is also found as part of pancytopenia; the main causes of pancytopenia are given in Table 9.1 on p. 143.

Agranulocytosis

The term agranulocytosis was originally used to refer to an acute febrile illness with necrotizing lesions of the mouth and throat associated with an extreme reduction or complete absence of neutrophil granulocytes in the peripheral blood. It is a rare condition and is now known to be caused by severe drug-induced neutropenia. The platelets and red cells are not affected. The first drug to be incriminated was amidopyrine, and although this compound is no longer prescribed, it is still available in some proprietary preparations in certain parts of the world. The prevalence of agranulocytosis in those taking the drug has been reported to be as high as 1%. Many other drugs will occasionally cause agranulocytosis. These include: some antithyroid drugs, especially thiouracil; certain tranquillizers such as chlorpromazine; some antibacterial drugs such as sulphonamides and chloramphenicol and several anti-inflammatory drugs, including phenylbutazone and gold salts. Many of these drugs may also cause aplastic anaemia. The mechanism of action of these drugs, when known, is either through an antigen-antibody reaction or through interference with one or

Table 7.1 Some causes of selective neutropenia.

Physiological
Neutropenia in Blacks

Certain drugs
Anti-inflammatory drugs: indomethacin, oxyphenbutazone,
    phenylbutazone, sodium aurothiomalate

Anti-bacterial drugs: chloramphenicol, co-trimoxazole
    (sulphamethoxazole-trimethoprim), other sulphonamides

Some anticonvulsants, antidiabetic drugs, antithyroid drugs,
    antimalarial drugs, tranquillizers, antidepressants and
    antihistamines

Infections
Bacterial: overwhelming pyogenic infections, brucellosis, typhoid,
    miliary tuberculosis

Some viral, protozoal and fungal infections

Immune neutropenia
SLE, Felty's syndrome, autoimmune neutropenia, neonatal alloimmune
    neutropenia, amidopyrine-induced agranulocytosis

Miscellaneous
Hypothyroidism, hypopituitarism, cyclical neutropenia, familial
    benign chronic neutropenia

more metabolic processes in neutrophil precursors (e.g. suppression of DNA synthesis by chlorpromazine).

Agranulocytosis should always be considered in a patient presenting with a severe infection of the throat and sometimes elsewhere, accompanied by profound weakness and exhaustion. The treatment is withdrawal of any suspected drug and use of appropriate antibiotics. The mortality rate is high; the prognosis is better if there are some white-cell precursors in the marrow than when these are absent.

Lymphocytopenia (lymphopenia)

Lymphocytopenia is seen after the administration of corticosteroids, following trauma or surgery, in many acute infections or after high-dose radiotherapy or therapy with cytotoxic drugs. It is also found in Cushing's syndrome, uraemia, SLE, sarcoidosis, Hodgkin's disease and in certain immunodeficiency syndromes, including AIDS.

LEUCOCYTOSIS

An increase in the absolute count of white blood cells, neutrophils, eosinophils, basophils, monocytes and lymphocytes above the normal range is described, respectively, as leucocytosis, neutrophil leucocytosis, eosinophil leucocytosis (eosinophilia), basophil leucocytosis, monocytosis and lymphocytosis.

Neutrophil leucocytosis

This is the most common abnormality of white blood cells encountered in clinical practice. The causes of neutrophil leucocytosis are many and are summarized in Table 7.2. An important cause is infection by pyogenic organisms. Here, the neutrophil counts are usually in the range 10 to 30 $\times$ 10^9/litre, but may be higher. In addition, there may be some neutrophil metamyelocytes and myelocytes and very occasional myeloblasts on the blood film ('shift to the left' or 'left shift'), the neutrophils may show toxic granulation or Döhle bodies or both, and the neutrophil alkaline phosphatase score is raised (also see p.109). Toxic granules are abnormally coarse, reddish-violet (azurophilic) granules which are diffusely distributed throughout the cytoplasm and Döhle bodies are 1–2 μm-long pale greyish-blue cytoplasmic inclusions, which are usually situated at the periphery of the cell (Romanowsky stain). A shift to the left, toxic granulation and Döhle bodies reflect accelerated neutrophil granulocytopoiesis and may be seen not only in acute infections but also in non-infective inflammatory states (e.g. severe burns), in normal pregnancy and in patients with various malignant neoplasms.

Whereas adults respond to acute bacterial infections with a neutrophil leucocytosis, young children may respond with a lymphocytosis.

The neutrophil leucocytosis seen after exercise, in emotional states, after the administration of adrenaline, after electric shocks and in patients with convulsions and paroxysmal tachycardia are caused by a rapid shift of neutrophils from the marginated to the circulating granulocyte pool (p. 12).

Eosinophil leucocytosis (eosinophilia)

Eosinophilia is usually caused by allergic disorders in the UK and other developed countries and by parasitic infestations in tropical countries. The parasites that provoke the highest eosinophil counts are metazoa which invade tissues. Some causes of eosinophilia are given in Table 7.3 (Beeson & Bass 1977).

Table 7.2   Causes of neutrophil leucocytosis.

Physiological
Neonates, exercise, emotion, pregnancy, parturition, lactation

Pathological
Acute infections: especially by pyogenic bacteria
Acute inflammation not caused by infections: surgery, burns, infarcts, crush injuries, rheumatoid arthritis, myositis, vasculitis
Acute haemorrhage and acute haemolysis
Metabolic: uraemia, diabetic ketoacidosis, gout, acute thyrotoxicosis
Non-haematological malignancies: carcinoma, lymphoma, melanoma
Chronic myeloproliferative disorders: chronic granulocytic leukaemia, polycythaemia rubra vera, myelofibrosis
Drugs: adrenaline, corticosteroids
Miscellaneous: convulsions, paroxysmal tachycardia, electric shock, post-neutropenic rebound neutrophilia, post-splenectomy

---

Table 7.3   Causes of eosinophilia.

Parasitic infestations: filariasis, hookworm, ascariasis,
   strongyloidiasis, schistosomiasis, toxocariasis, trichinosis, hydatid
   cyst, scabies
Allergic disorders: bronchial asthma, hay fever, allergic vasculitis,
   Stevens–Johnson syndrome, drug sensitivity (e.g. chlorpromazine,
   penicillin, sulphonamides)
Recovery from acute infection
Skin diseases: eczema, psoriasis, pemphigus, dermatitis herpetiformis
Pulmonary eosinophilia: Loeffler's syndrome (pulmonary infiltration with
   eosinophilia)
Hypereosinophilic syndrome
Polyarteritis nodosa
Leukaemias and chronic myeloproliferative disorders: chronic granulocytic
   leukaemia, eosinophilic leukaemia (rare)
Other malignant diseases: Hodgkin's disease, angioimmunoblastic
   lymphadenopathy, carcinoma (usually with metastases)

Hypereosinophilic syndrome

Very high eosinophil counts, sometimes accompanied by anaemia and thrombo-cytopenia are found in a disorder of uncertain aetiology named the hyper-eosinophilic syndrome. The clinical features of this disorder include fever, night sweats, weight loss, splenomegaly and damage to the heart, lungs and nervous system.

Cardiac damage is a characteristic feature. The lesions consist of areas of eosinophilic infiltration, muscle necrosis and fibrosis mainly affecting the endocardium and subendocardial myocardium; they have been attributed to the cytotoxic effects of a constituent of eosinophil granules. At least in some cases, the hypereosinophilic syndrome appears to be primarily a disease of the bone marrow and terminates in acute leukaemia.

Monocytosis and lymphocytosis

A high monocyte count ($>0.8 \times 10^9$/litre) is characteristic of certain bacterial infections, notably brucellosis, tuberculosis, typhoid fever and subacute bacterial endocarditis. Other conditions associated with a monocytosis are given in Table 7.4 (Maldonado & Hanlon 1965).

Lymphocytosis (greater than 3.5×10^9 lymphocytes/litre in adults) is the usual response to many viral infections. In infectious mononucleosis (see p. 107), the high lymphocyte count is associated with the presence of large, atypical mononuclear cells (which are activated T-lymphocytes). The one acute bacterial infection which is characteristically accompanied by very high lymphocyte counts, sometimes in excess of 50×10^9/litre, is whooping cough (pertussis). Many other acute bacterial infections, which cause neutrophil leucocytosis in adults, may provoke a lymphocytosis in infants and young children. The various causes of lymphocytosis are listed in Table 7.5.

Table 7.4   Causes of monocytosis.

Bacterial infections: tuberculosis, brucellosis, syphilis, subacute
    bacterial endocarditis, typhoid, recovery from acute infections
Protozoal infections: leishmaniasis, malaria, trypanosomiasis
Rickettsial infections: typhus, Rocky Mountain spotted fever
Myelodysplastic syndromes
Leukaemias: monocytic and myelomonocytic leukaemias, chronic granulocytic
    leukaemia
Other malignant diseases: Hodgkin's disease, carcinoma, malignant
    histiocytosis
Miscellaneous: ulcerative colitis, Crohn's disease

Table 7.5   Causes of lymphocytosis

Viral infections: infectious mononucleosis (glandular fever),
    cytomegalovirus infection, rubella, chicken pox, measles,
    mumps, influenza, infectious hepatitis
Bacterial infections: pertussis, other acute bacterial infections in
    infants and young children, tuberculosis, brucellosis, syphilis.
Chronic lymphocytic leukaemia
Lymphomas and Waldenström's macroglobulinaemia
Post-splenectomy (often temporary)

Infectious mononucleosis (glandular fever)

This is a usually benign infectious disease in which the epithelial cells of the
nasopharynx and B-lymphocytes are infected by the Epstein–Barr virus (EBV).
The virus is found in saliva, and transmission is by droplets or by kissing. The
incubation period is about 5–7 weeks. A high proportion of individuals become
infected early in childhood and about 90% of adults have EBV-related
antibodies. Most of those infected have subclinical or mild attacks; this is
particularly true of children. The syndrome of glandular fever is usually seen in
adolescents and young adults. The most common symptoms are malaise and
fatigue, sweats, sore throat and dysphagia, anorexia, nausea, headaches and
fever. Pharyngitis and follicular tonsillitis are often seen. In most cases, there is
bilateral cervical lymphadenopathy and in some cases there may also be
enlargement of axillary and inguinal glands. In about half the patients, there is
mild or moderate splenomegaly and in about 20%, there is slight hepatomegaly.
Some patients have periorbital oedema and a small number have a maculopap-
ular skin rash or jaundice. Very occasionally, there may be splenic rupture,
thrombocytopenic purpura, disseminated intravascular coagulation, autoimmune haemolytic anaemia (cold antibody with anti-i or, less often, anti-I
specificity), aplastic anaemia, liver failure, pericarditis, myocarditis or nervous
system involvement (Banatvala 1970; Pullen 1973).

   The two characteristic findings in the peripheral blood are an increase in the
absolute lymphocyte count above the upper limit of normal of 3.5×10^9/litre,
usually up to 10–20×10^9/litre, and the appearance of lymphocytes with
abnormal morphology, often described as atypical mononuclear cells (Fig. 7.1,
Plates 15,16). The morphology of these cells is variable and very similar to that

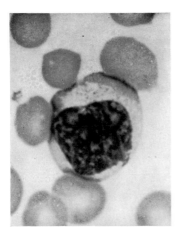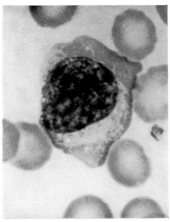

Fig. 7.1 Two atypical mononuclear cells from the blood film of a patient with glandular fever. As is commonly the case, the cytoplasmic basophilia is more marked at the periphery of the cell. Both cells are larger than normal lymphocytes.

of peripheral blood lymphocytes which have transformed following stimulation with mitogens *in vitro*. The abnormal cells are large, have moderately abundant very basophilic cytoplasm, possess a lobulated or indented nucleus with a relatively fine chromatin pattern and prominent nucleoli, and display a scalloped margin at points of contact with other cells on a blood film (Carter 1966). The atypical mononuclear cells are T-lymphocytes which are reacting against infected B-lymphocytes which have virus-encoded antigens on their surface (only B-cells have a receptor for EBV). Most of the infected B-cells are morphologically normal and the absolute B-lymphocyte count is increased.

In most patients with glandular fever, heterophile antibodies develop. These are antibodies formed in response to antigens of one species, which cross-react with antigens on the cells of other species. The most characteristic heterophile antibody agglutinates sheep and horse red cells and is absorbed by ox red cells but not by guinea pig kidney. The Paul–Bunnell test and other simpler tests for glandular fever are based on the detection of this antibody which develops in 80–90% of patients during the second and third weeks of the illness; the antibody declines and is usually undetectable after 2–3 months. Antibodies against proteins produced by the virus also appear at the same time and persist for years, giving lasting immunity.

LEUKAEMOID REACTIONS

Occasionally, patients are seen in whom the peripheral blood findings suggest at first sight that they could have leukaemia, but in reality the changes are an unusual response to some other disorder. The total white cell count is over 50×10^9/litre and the blood picture may resemble that seen in chronic granulocytic leukaemia (CGL) or chronic lymphocytic leukaemia. Leukaemoid reactions resembling acute leukaemia are rare but may be found in disseminated tuberculosis and in Down's syndrome (during the neonatal period).

In the type simulating CGL there are many immature white cells (myelocytes, promyelocytes and a few myeloblasts) in the peripheral blood. This abnormal reaction sometimes occurs as the result of severe infection, especially in children, and also in patients with malignant tumours, rapid haemolysis and burns. The following characteristics of granulocytic leukaemoid reactions help to distinguish them from chronic granulocytic leukaemia: the neutrophils may show toxic granulation and Döhle bodies (Plates 17, 18), the basophil and eosinophil counts are not raised, and the alkaline phosphatase score in the polymorphs is normal or increased, not reduced as in CGL.

Lymphocytic leukaemoid reactions may be seen as an 'excessive' response to infection, usually infectious mononucleosis and pertussis.

LEUCOERYTHROBLASTIC REACTION

The characteristic feature is the presence of a number of nucleated red cells (erythroblasts) as well as immature white cells (mainly myelocytes) in the peripheral blood film. The total white cell count may or may not be elevated. A leucoerythroblastic blood picture may be found when the bone marrow is infiltrated with malignant cells (carcinoma, lymphoma, myeloma, leukaemia), fibrous tissue (primary or secondary myelofibrosis) or storage cells (e.g. Gaucher's disease). It may also occur after severe haemorrhage and when there is marked haemolysis. A bone marrow aspiration often helps to establish the diagnosis.

MYELODYSPLASTIC SYNDROMES

This term is used to describe a group of conditions in which there is evidence of disordered maturation (dysplasia) in one or more of the myeloid cell lineages. Blood cell production from the dysplastic cell lineages is ineffective and, consequently, may lead to anaemia, thrombocytopenia or neutropenia. The population of dysplastic cells seems to represent an abnormal clone derived from a multipotent myeloid stem cell. The abnormal clone is stable for a variable period (sometimes for several years). It may, however, generate new clones associated with increasingly ineffective haemopoiesis, or increasing dysfunction of mature cells, or frankly malignant properties. The latter results in the haematological picture of acute myeloid leukaemia. In some patients, the myelodysplastic syndrome is a consequence of previous cytotoxic therapy or irradiation, but in most patients no aetiological factor is readily identifiable.

The majority of patients are elderly. In people over the age of 60 years, the incidence of myelodysplastic syndromes has been estimated to be six times that of acute myeloid leukaemia (Hamblin & Oscier 1987). Some patients are diagnosed incidentally as a consequence of having a blood count for an unrelated reason. Others present with symptoms referable to anaemia, thrombocytopenia or neutropenia and to functional abnormalities of neutrophils and platelets (i.e. lethargy and dyspnoea, spontaneous bruising and other haemorrhagic symptoms, or infections).

A variety of abnormalities may be seen on the blood film; often only a single abnormality may be found at diagnosis and others appear later. Abnormalities that may be found in the peripheral blood are: macrocytosis of red cells (not due

Table 7.6 FAB classification of myelodysplastic syndromes.

Syndrome	Peripheral blood	Bone marrow
Refractory anaemia*	Blasts <1%	Blasts <5%; ringed sideroblasts <15%
Refractory anaemia with ringed sideroblasts (primary acquired sideroblastic anaemia)	High MCV; dimorphic red cell picture	Blasts <5%; ringed sideroblasts >15%
Refractory anaemia with excess of blasts (RAEB)	Blasts <5%	Blasts 5–20%
Chronic myelomonocytic leukaemia (CMML)	Monocyte count >1.0 × 10^9/litre; granulocytes often increased; blasts <5%	Blasts <20%; promonocytes may be increased
RAEB in transformation	Blasts >5% or Auer rods present	Blasts 20–30% or Auer rods present

*Some patients who have neutropenia and/or thrombocytopenia without anaemia are classified with this category ('refractory cytopenia')

to B_{12} or folate deficiency), neutrophils with a reduced number of granules (Plate 19) or with the Pelger–Huet phenomenon (bi-lobed spectacle-like nuclei) (Plate 20) and abnormally large platelets. Abnormalities found in the bone marrow include: megaloblastic erythropoiesis (not due to B_{12} or folate deficiency), ringed sideroblasts, multinuclearity and irregularities of nuclear outline in erythroblasts and small megakaryocytes with abnormal nuclei. There may be chromosomal abnormalities, such as monosomy 5 or 7. In contrast to acute myeloid leukaemia, the blast cells account for less than 30% of nucleated marrow cells.

On the basis of the haematological findings, the French–American–British (FAB) cooperative group has classified the myelodysplastic syndromes into five categories (Bennett *et al.* 1982): the details of this classification are shown in Table 7.6. The syndrome of refractory anaemia with ringed sideroblasts carries a considerably better prognosis than the others, only a small proportion of cases developing acute leukaemia.

Patients are only treated when symptoms become troublesome. Management of the severe cytopenias is difficult and essentially supportive (e.g. platelet transfusions and appropriate antimicrobial treatment when necessary, regular transfusions of red cells). Drugs that may have some beneficial effect on the blood count include *cis*-retinoic acid and low doses of cytosine arabinoside. Once acute myeloid leukaemia develops, most patients die within a few months; the leukaemia responds poorly to therapy.

THE LEUKAEMIAS (GENERAL CONSIDERATIONS)

The leukaemias are malignant neoplasms of the precursors of blood cells; the malignant cells usually circulate in the blood and infiltrate tissues. Leukaemias are clonal disorders; that is, they arise from the malignant transformation usually of a single cell. In about 20% of cases of acute leukaemia and in chronic granulocytic leukaemia, the cell undergoing the transformation is probably a pluripotent stem cell (i.e. the cell which eventually gives rise to all types of blood cell, including lymphocytes). In other cases, the leukaemia seems to arise from a more mature progenitor cell which may be restricted to only 1–3 lines of differentiation. By repeated cell division, the transformed cell generates an expanding clone of malignant cells and their progeny. In general, leukaemic cells divide at a slower rate than normal cells and show absent or disturbed maturation.

Classification

There are four common varieties of leukaemia: acute lymphoblastic, acute myeloid, chronic lymphocytic and chronic granulocytic (chronic myeloid). The terms acute and chronic refer to the clinical course in untreated patients; those with acute leukaemia usually die within weeks or months and those with chronic leukaemias usually survive longer. This clinical subdivision of leukaemia corresponds with the degree of maturity of the predominant leukaemic cell type found in the bone marrow and blood, in that immature, blast-like cells predominate in many acute leukaemias and more mature cells predominate in chronic leukaemias. The predominant cell types found in the four common types of leukaemia are shown in Table 7.7. In the last decade, monoclonal antibodies against various cellular antigens and cytochemical techniques have been increasingly applied to characterize the leukaemic cells more finely and thus further to subdivide the acute leukaemias. One currently popular classification is based on the proposals of a French–American–British (FAB) cooperative group (Bennett et al. 1976, 1980). The details of such classifications of the acute leukaemias are given in Tables 7.8–7.10 in order to illustrate the heterogeneity in the cytology of the leukaemic cell clone found both in acute lymphoblastic and in acute myeloid leukaemia.

Aetiology of leukaemia

The aetiology of leukaemia is still under investigation. Studies with inbred strains of mice have shown that the susceptibility of a mouse to develop leukaemia is

Table 7.7   Predominant abnormal cell types in the major forms of leukaemia.

Type of leukaemia	Predominant leukaemic cell type in bone marrow and blood
Acute lymphoblastic	Lymphoblasts
Acute myeloid	Usually myeloblasts. Sometimes promyelocytes, monoblasts or promonocytes. Occasionally erythroblasts and, rarely, megakaryoblasts
Chronic lymphocytic	Lymphocytes
Chronic granulocytic (chronic myeloid)	Neutrophil myelocytes and metamyelocytes, and neutrophil granulocytes

Table 7.8   FAB classification of acute lymphoblastic leukaemia(L1–L3) (Bennett *et al.* 1976).

FAB category	Features of leukaemic lymphoblasts
L1	Small; scanty cytoplasm; uniform appearance
L2	Large; more cytoplasm; heterogeneous in size and shape
L3	Large; moderately abundant basophilic cytoplasm; cytoplasmic vacuolation; cells are similar to those in Burkitt's lymphoma

based on a complex interaction between its genetic make-up and other factors such as its age, hormonal and immunological status and the degree of exposure to radiation or to leukaemogenic chemicals or viruses. For example, some strains of mice (e.g. C3H) rarely develop leukaemia spontaneously even in old age but readily do so after X-irradiation. By contrast other strains (e.g. Ak) regularly develop leukaemia in old age. The development of leukaemia in humans also seems to depend on an interplay between multiple factors. Furthermore, leukaemogenesis seems to occur by a process involving multiple steps. The factors thought to be involved in human leukaemogenesis and the evidence in support of their involvement are discussed below.

Ionizing radiation

The evidence that ionizing radiation is leukaemogenic in humans is very good and is based on finding an increased incidence of leukaemia in:

Table 7.9   FAB classification of acute myeloid leukaemia (M1–M7) (Bennett *et al.* 1976, 1980).

FAB category	Features of the bone marrow
M1, myeloblastic leukaemia without maturation	Myeloblasts predominate, most show little or no maturation
M2, myeloblastic leukaemia with maturation	Myeloblasts predominate, some show maturation to and beyond promyelocyte stage
M3, promyelocytic leukaemia	Promyelocytes predominate and are often hypergranular
M4, myelomonocytic leukaemia	Evidence of both granulocytic and monocytic maturation; promonocytes plus monocytes >20% in blood or marrow
M5, monocytic leukaemia	Monoblasts or promonocytes predominate
M6, erythroleukaemia	Presence of a high proportion of erythroblasts, often with marked morphological abnormalities
M7, megakaryoblastic leukaemia	Megakaryoblasts or micromegakaryocytes prominent. May be associated with acute myelofibrosis

Table 7.10 Classification of acute lymphoblastic leukaemias based on immunological markers.

Category	Percentage of cases of childhood ALL	Phenotype of leukaemic cells/presumed cell of origin	Corresponding FAB category
T-ALL	15–20	Thymocytes	L1 and L2
pre-B-ALL	20	Pre-B cells (have cytoplasmic μ chains)	L1 and L2
B-ALL	1–2	Mature B cells (have surface membrane Ig)	L3 and L2
Common-ALL	50	Non-T, non-B ALL. c-ALL antigen positive. Probably corresponds to an early cell committed to the B cell lineage	L1 and L2
Null-ALL	8	Non-T, non-B-ALL. c-ALL antigen negative. Probably more immature than cells in c-ALL	L1 and L2

1 the survivors of nuclear bomb explosions at Hiroshima and Nagasaki (i.e. individuals receiving a single large dose of whole-body ionizing radiation);

2 patients with ankylosing spondylitis who had received repeated irradiation to the spine.

Several features of leukaemia that follows whole or partial body irradiation are worthy of note. These are:

1 there is a direct correlation between the dose of irradiation received and the risk of developing leukaemia;

2 only a proportion of heavily irradiated individuals develop leukaemia (e.g. only 1 in 60 of the heavily irradiated atomic bomb victims developed leukaemia over 12 years);

3 there is often a substantial latent period (the peak incidence occurs five years after exposure);

4 radiation induces acute and chronic myeloid leukaemia and acute lymphoblastic leukaemia but not chronic lymphocytic leukaemia.

The validity of the observation that there is an increased incidence of leukaemia in children born to mothers who have been submitted to diagnostic radiology during pregnancy has not yet been settled.

Chemicals

One of the factors involved in leukaemogenesis seems to be the exposure of the population to certain chemicals such as environmental pollutants and drugs. There is good evidence that benzene is both myelotoxic and leukaemogenic;

myelosuppression usually precedes the emergence of leukaemia. There is also some evidence from epidemiological studies implicating other petroleum products, paints and pesticides in the aetiology of leukaemia. Treatment with various antitumour agents such as procarbazine, melphalan, thio-TEPA, chlorambucil, and cyclophosphamide is associated with an increased risk of developing leukaemia. In the case of melphalan, chlorambucil and cyclophosphamide this increased risk is seen even in patients treated for non-malignant disorders.

Viruses

Viruses are involved in leukaemogenesis in mice, rats, chickens and cats. However, the only virus which has been implicated in human leukaemogenesis to date is the retrovirus HTLV-1 which can be isolated from patients with adult T-cell leukaemia/lymphoma. This rare type of leukaemia is endemic in a localized area in Japan, but clusters and isolated cases have been found elsewhere, mainly in Blacks in the West Indies and the USA. HTLV-1 does not carry an oncogene and does not selectively integrate near a proto-oncogene. It may produce a regulatory protein which affects the activity of cellular genes.

Genetic factors

Some of the evidence implicating genetic factors in human leukaemogenesis is not as straightforward as the evidence obtained from experiments on genetically pure strains of mice. For instance, it has been shown that following the development of acute leukaemia in one of a pair of identical twins, there is a 25% chance of the co-twin also doing so within weeks or months. Furthermore, there are a relatively small number of reports in which between two to four cases of leukaemia occurred in one or more generations of the same family. On first glance, these data may appear to indicate the operation of genetic factors. However, there is controversy as to whether the frequency with which two or more cases of leukaemia have been observed in the same family is greater than that which would be expected by chance. Furthermore, as families share a common environment, the data on leukaemia in twins and familial leukaemia do not necessarily indicate the operation of genetic factors in leukaemogenesis; they may equally indicate the operation of environmental factors. More definite evidence of the importance of genetic factors in human leukaemogenesis comes from a high incidence of acute myeloid leukaemia in patients with Down's syndrome, Fanconi's anaemia and Bloom's syndrome, all of which are associated with congenital chromosomal abnormalities. Various acquired chromosomal abnormalities are seen in leukaemias (e.g. the Philadelphia chromosome in chronic myeloid leukaemia) and the relevance of some of these, and of oncogenes, in leukaemogenesis is discussed below.

Oncogenes

The growth of normal cells is under the control of a number of cellular genes known as proto-oncogenes. The products of such genes and the ways in which they regulate normal cell proliferation have not yet been fully elucidated. Some proto-oncogenes seem to code for growth factors or transmembrane growth factor receptors. Others code for proteins involved in the transduction of signals

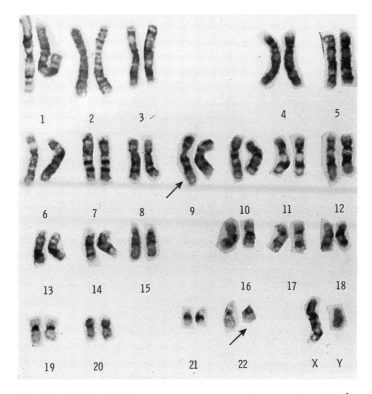

Fig. 7.2   G-R banded chromosome preparation from a male with Ph[1]-positive chronic granulocytic leukaemia. A portion of the chromosome from the long arm of one of the No. 22 pair has been translocated to the long arm of one of the No. 9 pair (both affected positions arrowed). (Reproduced with permission from Galton 1982)

from growth factor receptors at the cell surface to intracytoplasmic and intranuclear biochemical reactions regulating cell proliferation. There is evidence that in malignant cells, one or other of a number of genetic alterations affect proto-oncogenes which activate them into oncogenes (i.e. genes implicated in the generation of malignant change). In theory, activation of proto-oncogenes may be involved both in tumour initiation and in tumour progression (i.e. the evolution of the mutant clone, including the acquisition of malignant characteristics). The alterations known to activate proto-oncogenes include point mutations, insertion of viral genomes exerting transcriptional control near them, gene amplification (i.e. the generation of multiple gene copies) resulting in overexpression, and translocation into an actively transcribed locus. Recently, activation of certain oncogenes has been reported in some human leukaemias and lymphomas. For example, the formation of the Philadelphia chromosome in virtually all cases of chronic granulocytic leukaemia and in 5–25% of cases of acute lymphoblastic leukaemia is associated with the activation of the *abl* proto-oncogene. The Philadelphia chromosome (Fig. 7.2) is formed by translocation of part of the long arm of chromosome 22 to the long arm of chromosome 9 and this change is designated t9; 22 or, more precisely, t (9q + ;

22q –). The break point on chromosome 22 (situated in a breakpoint cluster region, BCR) is joined to the 3′ end of the *abl* gene on chromosome 9 and this results in a BCR-*abl* fusion gene and the consequent synthesis of a BCR-*abl* fusion protein. The gene product of the *abl* gene is a cytoplasmic tyrosine kinase which catalyses the phosphorylation of tyrosine and this phosphorylation seems to influence cell growth. The BCR-*abl* fusion protein formed in chronic myeloid leukaemia has altered tyrosine kinase activity. Examples of oncogene activation in human leukaemias are given in Table 7.11. Interestingly, point mutations in the N-*ras* proto-oncogenes have been reported not only in the acute leukaemias but also in some patients with the pre-leukaemic conditions known as the myelodysplastic syndromes (p. 109). Proto-oncogene activation has also been studied in detail in Burkitt's lymphoma; this is a high-grade B-cell lymphoma, not a leukaemia(p. 154). Here, translocation events juxtapose the *myc* gene on chromosome 8 next to the heavy chain locus on chromosome 14 [t(8;14)], or, less frequently, the k light chain locus on chromosome 2 [t(2;8)] or the λ light chain locus on chromosome 22 [t(8;22)].

It is possible that both chemical leukaemogens and leukaemogenic viruses can activate proto-oncogenes.

Table 7.11   Some oncogenes involved in human leukaemias.

Disease	Proto-oncogene	Proto-oncogene protein	Event activating proto-oncogene	Prevalence of activation (%)	Effects of activation on cell function
CGL	abl	Cytoplasmic tyrosine kinase	t(9;22), BCR on chromosome 22 translocated into abl on chromosome 9	100	BCR-abl fusion protein (210kD) with altered tyrosine kinase activity
ALL (B-cell)	abl	Cytoplasmic tyrosine kinase	t(9;22), BCR breakpoint differs from above	5–25	BCR-abl fusion protein (190kD)
ALL (B-cell)	N–ras	GTP-binding proteins involved in signal transduction	Point mutation	15	Mutant N-ras protein
AML	N–ras, K–ras, H–ras	GTP-binding proteins involved in signal transduction	Point mutation	25	Mutant ras protein
ALL (T-cell)	myc	Located in nucleus, function uncertain	t(8;14), myc on chromosome 8 translocated to T-cell receptor gene on chromosome 14	10–20	myc gene expression deregulated

CGL = chronic granulocytic leukaemia, ALL = acute lymphoblastic leukaemia, AML = acute myeloid leukaemia, t = chromosomal translocation, BCR = breakpoint cluster region on chromosome 22, including breakpoints involved in formation of Philadelphia chromosome.

Features common to all leukaemias

There are a number of features that are found in all the leukaemias. These are:

1   infiltration and replacement of normal bone marrow with leukaemic cells which causes anaemia, neutropenia and thrombocytopenia;

2   infiltration of other tissues and organs with leukaemic cells;

3   an increase in the basal metabolic rate when the tumour mass is large, leading to excessive sweating and loss of weight.

The most common clinical manifestations of leukaemia are related to the bone marrow infiltration. Thus, anaemia causes lassitude, weakness and shortness of breath and the neutropenia, which is aggravated by cytotoxic therapy, causes bacterial infections (pneumonia and septicaemia). The thrombocytopenia leads to abnormal bleeding.

Gram-negative infections predominate, the patient's own intestinal floral often being the source of septicaemias. The organisms are usually *Escherichia coli*, Klebsiella or *Pseudomonas aeruginosa*. Gram-positive infections (e.g. with *Staphylococcus aureus*) also occur and infections with unusual skin organisms such as *Staphylococcus epidermidis* may be seen consequent on the use of long-term indwelling catheters. When cytotoxic therapy causes marked immunosuppression, opportunistic infections (i.e. infections rarely seen in immunologically normal individuals) may occur with organisms such as *Candida*, *Aspergillus* and *Pneumocystis carinii*. Immunosuppression may also be associated with generalised and fulminant infections with viruses such as *herpes simplex* and *herpes zoster*.

The haemorrhagic manifestations often consist of purpura, epistaxis, bleeding from the gums and spontaneous bruising. Less commonly, bleeding may occur into other organs such as the nervous system, eye and internal ear.

The extent and nature of extramedullary tissue infiltration varies with both the type of leukaemia and the stage of progression of the disease. For example, whereas infiltration of lymph nodes is a common feature of the late stages of chronic lymphocytic leukaemia, it is unusual in acute myeloid leukaemia.

THE ACUTE LEUKAEMIAS

Both acute lymphoblastic leukaemia (ALL) and acute myeloid leukaemia (AML) occur at all ages. However, ALL is the most common type of acute leukaemia in children and AML is the most common type in adults. The incidence of ALL is 1–2 per 100,000 population per year; the age distribution shows a distinct peak at 3–4 years. The incidence of AML is low in children and rises with age, increasing from under two cases per 100 000 population per year in young adults to about 10–20 cases per 100 000 per year over the age of 65 years.

Clinical features

The patient is usually ill, with symptoms present for only a few days or weeks. The most common findings are pallor, fever, various infections and abnormal bleeding. In cases of acute promyelocytic leukaemia (M3), the haemorrhagic manifestations may be particularly severe due to activation of the fibrinolytic and coagulation systems by substances released from cytoplasmic granules. Painful, tender bones are frequently seen in ALL and cause affected children to limp.

There may be some enlargement of the liver, spleen and lymph nodes, although these findings are often absent in AML. Particularly in acute myelomonocytic leukaemia (M4) and acute monocytic leukaemia (M5), infiltration of the gums (Fig. 7.3) and skin may be seen. In T-ALL a mediastinal mass due to thymic enlargement is often found. Symptoms due to meningeal infiltration (headache, nausea and vomiting, visual disturbances) are rare at presentation but often develop during the course of acute leukaemia, and particularly of ALL, especially when CNS therapy is not given. Testicular infiltration is also common in treated cases of ALL.

Peripheral blood and bone marrow

A normochromic normocytic anaemia and thrombocytopenia are common. The concentration of white cells in the peripheral blood is usually increased, but this is not an essential feature of leukaemia. About one-third of patients with acute leukaemia have white-cell counts within or even below the normal range ($4–10 \times 10^9$/litre) during some stage of the disease, and the remainder have white-cell counts which usually fall in the range $10–50 \times 10^9$/litre). The neutrophil count is reduced, often markedly.

In the majority of cases of ALL, a variable proportion of the nucleated cells in the peripheral blood are lymphoblasts. In most patients, the blasts are small, have little cytoplasm, and are uniform in appearance (FAB category L1) (Plate 21), but in others they are larger, with more cytoplasm (L2 and L3; see Table 7.8 and Plate 22). The blood film in AML almost always contains variable numbers of myeloblasts (Fig. 7.4, Plates 23–25). In general, myeloblasts are larger, have more cytoplasm, and are more pleomorphic than lymphoblasts. Furthermore, a proportion of the myeloblasts may contain small numbers of azurophilic cytoplasmic granules, thus indicating their myeloid lineage (Plate 23). Some of the morphological, cytochemical and immunochemical features

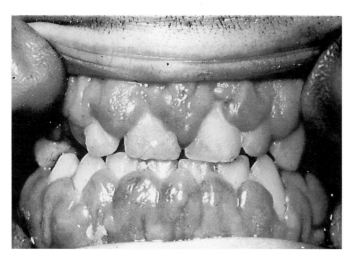

Fig. 7.3 Infiltration of gums by leukaemic cells (monoblasts) in a case of acute monocytic leukaemia.

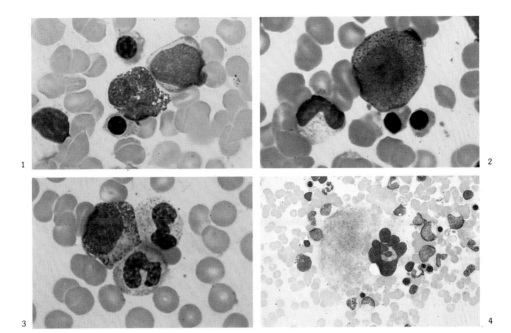

Plates 1–4 Haemopoietic cells from a smear of normal bone marrow (May–Grünwald–Giemsa stain). (1) Myeloblast, eosinophil granulocyte and two late polychromatic normoblasts. (2) Neutrophil promyelocyte, neutrophil metamyelocyte and two late polychromatic normoblasts. (3) Neutrophil myelocyte and two neutrophil metamyelocytes. (4) Mature megakaryocyte with granular cytoplasm; this polyploid cell is very large when compared with surrounding diploid bone marrow cells of various types.

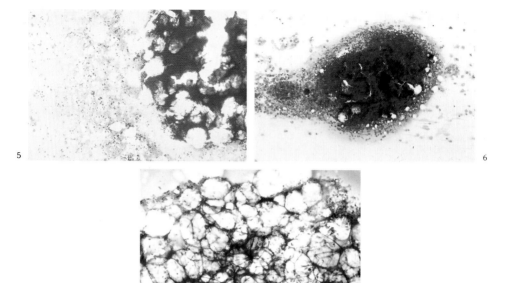

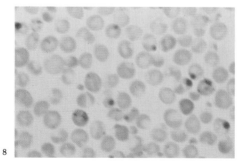

Plates 5–7 Different degrees of cellularity of marrow fragments in bone marrow smears from adults with three different disorders (May–Grünwald–Giemsa stain). (5) *Normocellular*: about half the volume of the fragment consists of haemopoietic cells (areas staining blue) and the remainder consists of rounded, pale-staining, fat cells; (6) *Markedly hypercellular*: virtually all the fat cells are replaced by haemopoietic cells. (7) *Markedly hypocellular*: there are only a few residual haemopoietic cells, most of the fragment consisting of fat cells.

Plate 8 Large, rounded, darkly-staining, membrane-bound Heinz bodies in the red cells of a splenectomized patient with HbH disease (supravital staining with methyl violet). Similar inclusions of denatured haemoglobin may also be found in G6PD-deficient patients exposed to oxidant substances. The Plate also shows two reticulocytes.

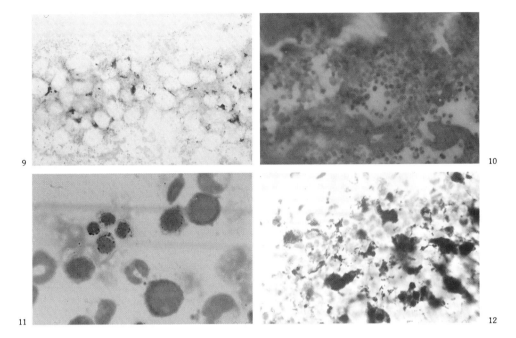

9

10

11

12

Plates 9–12 Bone marrow smears stained by Perls' acid ferrocyanide method for haemosiderin. (9) Marrow fragment containing normal quantities of storage iron. (10) Marrow fragment from a patient with iron deficiency anaemia showing an absence of storage iron. (11) Ringed sideroblasts from a patient with primary acquired sideroblastic anaemia. (12) Marrow fragment from a chronically-transfused patient with aplastic anaemia, showing a gross excess of storage iron.

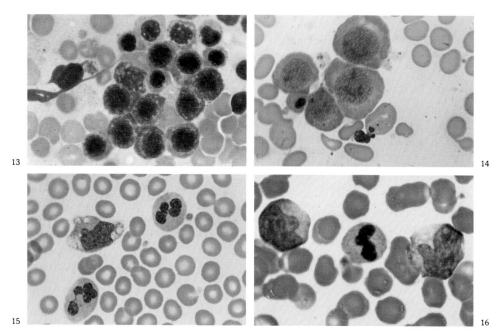

13   14

15   16

Plates 13–16 (13) Clump of early and late polychromatic normoblasts from the marrow of a patient with erythroid hyperplasia secondary to an autoimmune haemolytic anaemia. (14) Four early polychromatic megaloblasts and two late megaloblasts from the marrow of an untreated patient with pernicious anaemia. When compared with the early polychromatic normoblasts in Plate 13, the early polychromatic megaloblasts are larger and have more delicate, sieve-like nuclei containing much smaller particles of condensed chromatin. (15) A monocyte and two neutrophil granulocytes from a normal blood film. The monocyte has pale, greyish-blue, vacuolated cytoplasm. (16) Two atypical mononuclear cells and a neutrophil granulocyte from the blood film of a patient with glandular fever. Although the atypical mononuclear cells are similar in size to the monocyte in Plate 15, their cytoplasm is much more basophilic and not vacuolated. (May–Grünwald–Giemsa stain.)

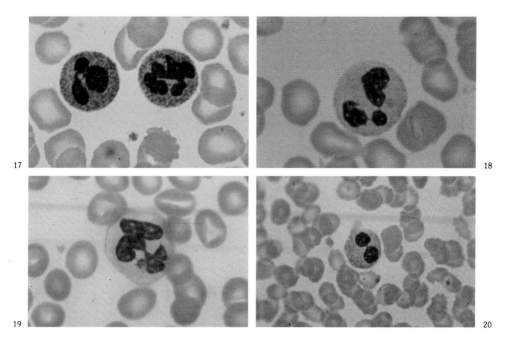

17

18

19

20

Plates 17–20 (17) Toxic granulation in two neutrophil granulocytes from a patient with an infection. (18) Round, pale-blue Döhle body near the nucleus of a neutrophil granulocyte from a patient with extensive burns. Döhle bodies may also be oval or rod-shaped and are more frequently seen at the periphery than at the centre of the cell. (19) Hypogranular neutrophil granulocyte from a patient with a myelodysplastic syndrome. (20) Neutrophil granulocyte from a heterozygote for the inherited Pelger–Huet anomaly. The nucleus is bilobed, spectacle-like and has markedly condensed chromatin. In heterozygotes for this asymptomatic condition, 50–70% of neutrophil granulocytes show these changes. Similar abnormalities may be found in some neutrophil granulocytes, as an acquired condition, in the myelodysplastic syndromes. (May–Grünwald–Giemsa stain.)

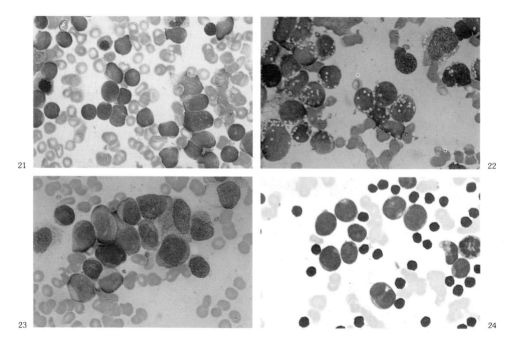

Plates 21–24 Bone marrow smears from patients with acute leukaemia showing infiltration by leukaemic blast cells (May–Grünwald–Giemsa stain). (21) Acute lymphoblastic leukaemia, FAB category L1. (22) Acute lymphoblastic leukaemia, FAB category L3; see Table 7.8 on p. 112 for differences from L1 and note prominent cytoplasmic vacuolation. (23) Acute myeloid leukaemia, FAB category M2; note that some of the leukaemic myeloblasts have azurophilic cytoplasmic granules. (24) Combination of acute myeloid leukaemia and chronic lymphocytic leukaemia in the same patient. Note the presence of two populations of leukaemic cells, the myeloblasts of acute myeloid leukaemia and the much smaller lymphocytes of chronic lymphocytic leukaemia.

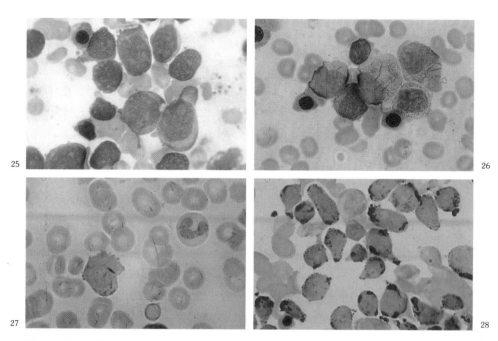

25

26

27

28

Plates 25–28 Bone marrow smears from patients with acute leukaemia. (25) Acute myeloid leukaemia (FAB category M1); the leukaemic myeloblasts are shown at higher magnification than in Plate 23. (26) Myeloblasts of acute myeloid leukaemia showing several Auer rods. These are azurophilic needle-shaped or rod-shaped intracytoplasmic inclusions which are exclusively found in some of the leukaemic myeloblasts of a small proportion of patients with acute myeloid leukaemia or chronic myeloid leukaemia in blast cell transformation. (27) Leukaemic myeloblasts stained with Sudan black, showing positive staining of Auer rods. (28) Acute lymphoblastic leukaemia; the smear has been stained by the Periodic acid–Schiff reaction and shows large positively-stained blocks in the cytoplasm of the leukaemic lymphoblasts.

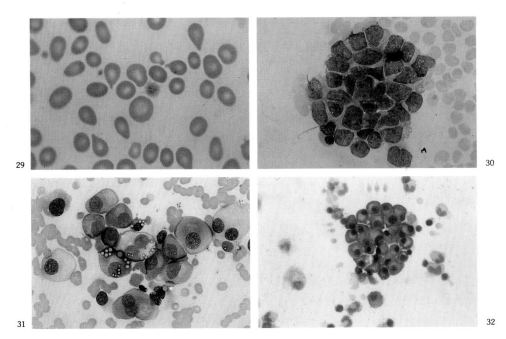

Plates 29–32 (29) Peripheral blood film of a patient with idiopathic myelofibrosis showing several tear-drop-shaped poikilocytes and an abnormally large platelet. (30) Clump of metastatic tumour cells in a marrow smear. (31) Marrow smear from a patient with multiple myeloma. (32) Marrow smear showing myeloma cells reacting with antibody against λ-chains; the reaction was demonstrated using an immuno-alkaline phosphatase (APAAP) method. The cells did not react with antibody against κ-chains and were, therefore, monoclonal in origin. The serum contained an IgD λ paraprotein.

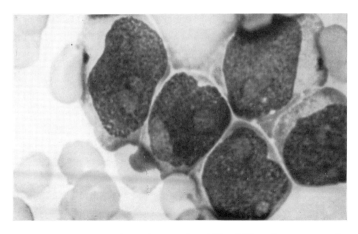

Fig. 7.4 Myeloblasts from the peripheral blood film of a patient with acute myeloid leukaemia. The diameters of these myeloblasts are several times those of adjacent red cells. Their nuclei appear finely stippled and have more than one nucleolus.

that are used to distinguish between leukaemic myeloblasts and lymphoblasts are summarized in Table 7.12. In addition to myeloblasts, other abnormal cells may be found in the blood in AML. These include promyelocytes, myelocytes, agranular neutrophils, neutrophils with the acquired Pelger anomaly (Plate 20), cells of the monocytic series, erythroblasts and megakaryoblasts (see Table 7.7).

Table 7.12 Some differences between leukaemic lymphoblasts and myeloblasts.

	Lymphoblast	Myeloblast
Nucleoli	1–2	2–5
Amount of cytoplasm	Usually scanty	Moderate
Auer rods	Absent	Sometimes present (Plates 26,27)
Sudan black	Negative	Positive
Peroxidase	Negative	Positive
PAS	Positive; large blocks or coarse granules of stained material against a negative background (Plate 28)	Negative or diffuse tinge ± fine granules
Chloroacetate esterase	Negative	Usually positive
Terminal deoxynucleotidyl transferase (TdT)	Positive	Usually negative
Immunological markers	T-cell lineage markers (e.g. CD2) or B-cell lineage markers (e.g. CD19)	Myeloid lineage markers (e.g. CD13 or CD33)

In occasional patients with acute leukaemia, blast cells may be either absent or difficult to find in the peripheral blood at presentation; such patients are described as having aleukaemic leukaemia.

In both ALL and AML, the bone marrow is usually very hypercellular. In ALL, it is extensively infiltrated with lymphoblasts and lymphocytes. Differences in the morphology of lymphoblasts in the different FAB categories (L1-L3) are given in Table 7.8. In AML, more than 30% of the nucleated marrow cells are leukaemic blasts (usually myeloblasts), or more than 50% are myeloblasts plus promyelocytes. The special cytological features of the bone marrow in different FAB categories of AML (M1 — M7) are shown in Table 7.9.

About 25% of adults and 1–4% of children with ALL have the Ph[1] chromosome in their blast cells. Since some patients with chronic granulocytic leukaemia (CGL) may undergo a lymphoblastic transformation and some patients with ALL may develop CGL, it seems that the cell of origin of Ph[1]-positive ALL may be a pluripotent stem cell (i.e. a cell which gives rise both to the lymphoid stem cells and the multipotent myeloid stem cells). Ph[1]-negative cases of ALL may have other non-random chromosomal abnormalities. Chromosome abnormalities are also common in the marrow cells of patients with AML and certain abnormalities are uniquely associated with some FAB categories.

Treatment

This is based on combinations of cytotoxic drugs and, in some circumstances, allogeneic or autologous bone marrow transplantation. Different cytotoxic regimes are used in ALL and AML. About half of all children with common ALL can be cured with drug schedules including prednisolone and vincristine. By contrast, cytotoxic drugs are much less effective in adults with ALL and in AML. The modes of action of some of the drugs used in the treatment of acute leukaemia are given in Table 7.13. Attempts at killing all leukaemic cells by whole body irradiation plus intensive chemotherapy have to be followed by marrow transplantation.

Acute lymphoblastic leukaemia (ALL)

Therapy with red cell and platelet transfusions and antibiotics may be necessary at presentation. A standard regime for remission induction in children is prednisolone, vincristine and L-asparaginase. These drugs induce a complete haematological remission in 93% of cases overall; the remission rate is nearly 100% in c-ALL but is lower in T-ALL, B-ALL and null-ALL. The same drug regime induces fewer remissions and shorter disease-free survival in adults than in children. The inclusion of additional drugs (e.g. an anthracycline) in the induction regime improves the remission rate in children with adverse prognostic features and in adults, but may lead to substantial marrow suppression. If severe marrow suppression occurs, intensive support of the type used in AML (see p. 121) will be needed. Patients are also treated with intrathecal methotrexate with or without cranial irradiation to reduce the risk of their developing meningeal leukaemia. In addition, maintenance therapy is carried out for a prolonged period (e.g. 2–3 years) with various cytotoxic drugs in an attempt to

Table 7.13 Modes of action of some cytotoxic drugs used in acute leukaemia.

Drugs	Mode of action
Prednisolone	Uncertain
Vincristine	Blocks formation of microtubules of the mitotic spindle
L-asparaginase	Starves cells of arginine
Methotrexate	Inhibits dihydrofolate reductase and, consequently, thymidylate synthesis
Daunorubicin, hydroxydaunorubicin (Adriamycin)	Intercalate between DNA base pairs and inhibit DNA synthesis
Cytosine arabinoside	Pyrimidine analogue; becomes incorporated into DNA and blocks transcription
Thioguanine, 6-mercaptopurine	Purine analogues; become incorporated into DNA and block transcription

kill all residual leukaemic cells. There may also be a place for a short period or periods of intensive chemotherapy to consolidate the remission. With this type of treatment, about 50% of children with ALL attain long-term disease-free survival and many of these are considered to be cured. With intensive therapy, the proportion of adults attaining long-term disease-free survival is about 35%. A second remission may be induced by chemotherapy in patients who relapse but is short-lived. Those who relapse after a first remission should be considered for transplantation if a second remission can be induced.

Some authorities consider that patients with a white-cell count greater than 100×10^9/litre at presentation, those aged between 14 and 45 years and those with B-ALL, all of whom have a relatively poor prognosis, should be considered for allogeneic bone marrow transplantation in the first remission. However, Butturini & Gale (1989) have recently argued that, even in these patients, comparable leukaemia-free long-term survival could be obtained by transplantation during the second remission.

Acute myeloid leukaemia (AML)

A combination of drugs is used to induce remission; drug and dosage schedules are being revised continuously according to empirical observations on their efficacy. An effective combination consists of daunorubicin and cytosine arabinoside, with or without a third drug such as thioguanine. With this type of treatment, prolonged marrow hypoplasia occurs; this is followed by a complete haematological remission in 60% of cases. The drugs cause severe neutropenia and immunosuppression. Intensive support is required during the phase of marrow hypoplasia, including red cell and platelet transfusions and prophylactic oral antibiotics (to minimize the risk of septicaemia, particularly from the patient's own gut flora). If significant fever develops in a patient with a neutrophil count of less than 0.5×10^9/litre, empiric antibiotic treatment (e.g.

with gentamicin and piperacillin intravenously) should be started immediately after taking blood for culture. Successful induction of remission is usually consolidated by a further course or courses of cytotoxic therapy. Maintenance therapy is of doubtful value and is not always given. The median duration of remission has slowly increased over the years and is now about two years, but disease-free long-term survival is seen only in 20% of cases.

Allogeneic bone marrow transplantation should be considered in appropriate cases during the first remission. About 40% of patients transplanted in first remission are free of disease at 3 years; since relapse of leukaemia is rare after this time, many of these patients are probably cured. An equally effective strategy may be to transplant at first relapse or during a second remission (Butturini & Gale 1989). The problems associated with allogeneic transplantation are: failure to engraft or rejection following engraftment (rare); graft-versus-host disease and recurrence of leukaemia. Autologous marrow transplantation can be considered in older patients (who tolerate allogeneic transplantation poorly) and in those without a suitable donor, although its efficacy is unproven as yet. Marrow is aspirated and cryopreserved during the first remission. When the patient relapses, chemoradiotherapy is given and the stored marrow is used to reconstitute haemopoiesis, sometimes after purging residual leukaemic cells *in vitro* using a variety of techniques.

CHRONIC LYMPHOCYTIC LEUKAEMIA (CLL)

This is the commonest form of chronic leukaemia, with an incidence of 2–3 per 100 000 population per year. The male: female ratio is 2:1. CLL is rare before the age of 35; over this age, its incidence rises progressively with increasing age. In 98% of cases the malignant clone consists of B-lymphocytes (B-CLL) and in the remainder it consists of T-lymphocytes (T-CLL). Symptoms are not only due to infiltration of the bone marrow and other tissues by the malignant cells, but also to a disturbance of both humoral and cellular immunity. There is a reduction in the number of normal B-lymphocytes resulting in a reduced ability to make antibodies. In addition, there is an increase of suppressor T cells and a reduction of helper T cells which probably accounts for the impairment of cell-mediated immunity. Autoimmune phenomena develop in some cases.

Clinical features

Initially CLL is asymptomatic and it is not uncommon for the disease to be discovered accidentally while carrying out a peripheral blood examination for some unrelated reason. Later, the patients are mildly or severely ill and give a history of symptoms that have been present for several months or years. The commonest presenting symptoms are loss of energy, tiredness and shortness of breath. Some patients notice enlargement of superficial lymph nodes. Early in the course of the disease no abnormalities are found on clinical examination. Subsequently, enlargement of the superficial lymph nodes, hepatomegaly and splenomegaly are found. Splenic enlargement is less marked than in chronic myeloid leukaemia, the spleen being rarely enlarged below the level of the umbilicus.

Impairment of humoral immunity and severe neutropenia are present in the later stages of the disease and may cause pneumococcal pneumonia and meningitis and other bacterial infections. The impaired cellular immunity increases susceptibility to infection with *Mycobacterium tuberculosis* and with certain fungi (candida, cryptococcus) and viruses (herpes zoster, herpes simplex and vaccinia).

Other less common findings include infiltration of the tonsils or skin and Mikulicz's syndrome (enlargement of lachrymal and salivary glands).

Peripheral blood and bone marrow

The essential finding in the peripheral blood is an increase in the lymphocyte count, which may be anywhere between 3.5×10^9/litre and over 300×10^9/litre; it is usually greater than 15×10^9/litre (Fig. 7.5). Most of the lymphocytes are mature small lymphocytes (Fig. 7.6). A characteristic feature of the blood film in CLL is the presence of a number of 'smear cells' or 'smudge cells'. These result from an increased mechanical fragility of the malignant lymphocytes which are consequently disrupted and squashed during the preparation of blood films. Even when the lymphocytosis is not marked (e.g. below 15×10^9/litre), the diagnosis of CLL can be made by demonstrating that the population of lymphocytes is monoclonal (e.g. by showing that the surface membrane immunoglobulin is of only one light chain type).

Normochromic normocytic anaemia, thrombocytopenia and neutropenia, all due to marrow infiltration, are seen in the later stages of the disease. A positive direct antiglobulin test is found in about 10% of cases and some of these show a mild to severe autoimmune haemolytic anaemia with jaundice, a high reticulocyte count and spherocytosis (p. 48). Some patients may develop autoimmune thrombocytopenic purpura.

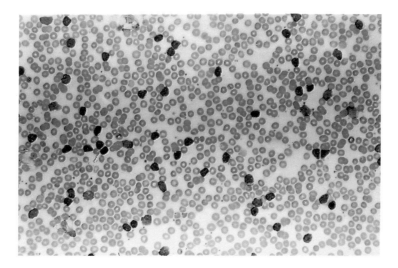

Fig. 7.5 Blood film of a patient with chronic lymphocytic leukaemia who had a markedly increased lymphocyte count of 135×10^9/litre.

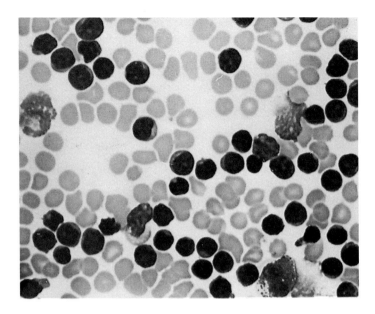

Fig. 7.6 Blood film of another patient with chronic lymphocytic leukaemia shown at higher magnification than in Fig. 7.5 (lymphocyte count 300 × 10⁹/litre). There is a marked increase in mature small lymphocytes with scanty cytoplasm and densely-staining nuclei. There are also some smear cells.

About 50% of patients with CLL have subnormal 1gG, IgA and IgM levels.

Bone marrow aspirates are hypercellular and show varying degrees of infiltration, mainly with mature small lymphocytes but also with larger lymphoid cells. Normal haemopoietic cells may be reduced in number.

Progression of changes in CLL

Dameshek (1967) considered CLL to be a condition in which there was a gradual accumulation of inactive but long-lived lymphocytes. With this concept in mind, Rai et al (1975) analysed 125 patients and found that four stages in the disease can be characterized, progression from one stage to the next being associated with a shorter life span (Table 7.14). Thus, at stage 0 there was only lymphocytosis (>15 × 10⁹/litre) and more than 40% of bone marrow cells were lymphocytes; this stage was associated with a median survival of some 10–20 years from the time the stage was diagnosed, the longest lived patient was still alive after 32 years. In stage I, the lymph nodes became palpable and the median survival from then onward was 8 years. Stage II was characterized by lymphocytosis with enlargement of the liver or spleen or both, and the median survival was 6 years. Stage III was characterized by lymphocytosis and anaemia (haemoglobin concentration, <11 g/dl) and stage IV by lymphocytosis and thrombocytopenia (platelet count, <100 × 10⁹/litre); the median survival at these stages was 1–2 years.

Death is often due to causes unrelated to the CLL but may be due to infection complicating neutropenia and immunodeficiency. Rarely, death occurs as a result of malignant transformation. This may be of one of two types:

Table 7.14 Staging of chronic lymphocytic leukaemia. The asterisk sign (*) gives the essential feature indicating the stage reached.

Stage	Lymphocytosis (blood and marrow)	Enlarged lymph nodes	Enlarged spleen and liver	Anaemia	Thrombo-cytopenia	Median survival (years)
0	*	−	−	−	−	10–20
I	+	*	−	−	−	8
II	+	+ or −	*	−	−	6
III	+	+ or −	+ or −	*	−	1–2
IV	+	+ or −	+ or −	+ or −	*	1–2

1 *prolymphocytic transformation*, in which many of the malignant cells in the blood and marrow have the morphology of prolymphocytes rather than small lymphocytes;
2 *blastic transformation (Richter's syndrome)*, which starts at one site and is manifest by a selective increase in the rate of tumour growth at that site. Eventually, blast cells appear in the circulation and a blood picture resembling that of acute leukaemia results.

Treatment

It is still not certain whether long-term treatment from the time of diagnosis prolongs survival. Consequently, treatment is usually aimed at alleviating symptoms when they develop and at improving bone marrow function when evidence of failure is detected. No treatment is given for stage 0. Stages I and II are only treated if there is bulky lymphadenopathy or if splenomegaly causes discomfort or 'hypersplenism'. The remaining stages are associated with impairment of normal haemopoiesis and must be treated, as must patients with autoimmune haemolytic anaemia.

Most patients respond to the alkylating agent, chlorambucil, either given continuously or in intermittent courses. Cyclophosphamide, another alkylating agent, is also effective.

Prednisolone causes a rapid temporary reduction in tumour mass but should not be given for prolonged periods as it increases the chance of infection in an already immunocompromised patient. It is useful in the initial management of autoimmune haemolytic anaemia and of marked marrow failure.

Local radiotherapy is effective in shrinking selected masses of tumour tissue which are causing problems by virtue of their size. It is also of value in the management of hypersplenism when the splenomegaly does not respond to chemotherapy.

Infections should be treated vigorously when they occur. Patients with recurrent infections are helped by regular intravenous gammaglobulin therapy.

CHRONIC GRANULOCYTIC LEUKAEMIA, CGL (CHRONIC MYELOID LEUKAEMIA)

The incidence of this form of chronic leukaemia is about 1 per 100 000 population per year. The disease is rare in children; its incidence in adults rises steadily with increasing age. The Philadelphia chromosome (p. 115) is present in over 95% of the cases, not only in neutrophil precursors but also in erythroblasts, megakaryocytes and B-lymphocytes. The malignant clone appears to arise from a pluripotent haemopoietic stem cell.

Clinical features

Most patients are symptomatic at the time of diagnosis. Common symptoms are low-grade fever, anorexia, weight loss and night sweats (due to a raised metabolic rate), lassitude, dyspnoea and palpitations (due to anaemia), discomfort over the left side of the abdomen (due to massive splenomegaly) and bruising and other haemorrhagic manifestations (due to abnormalities in the number and function of platelets). Rarer symptoms seen in patients with WBC >500 × 10^9/litre are headaches, dizziness, tinnitus, deafness, ataxia and even coma; these result from impairment of cerebral blood flow due to increased blood viscosity as well as from vascular obstruction by leucocytes. Priapism is also seen occasionally and may have the same basis. Gout and uric acid stones may result from hyperuricaemia due to increased nucleic acid turnover.

Peripheral blood and bone marrow

The blood count often shows a normochromic normocytic anaemia. The white cell count is elevated, usually to between 50 × 10^9/litre and 400 × 10^9/litre. The platelet count is often high, but may be normal or low. Most of the white cells consist of neutrophil granulocytes, metamyelocytes and myelocytes (see Figs. 7.6 and 7.7). Blast cells account for a relatively small proportion of the leucocytes. There is virtually always an increase in the absolute basophil count and, commonly, also an increase in the absolute eosinophil and monocyte counts. Megakaryocytes may be seen in the blood film. The neutrophil alkaline

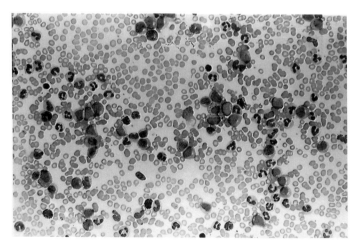

Fig. 7.7 Blood film of a patient with chronic granulocytic leukaemia. The total white cell count is markedly increased (200 × 10^9/litre) and the majority of the white cells consists of neutrophil granulocytes, metamyelocytes and myelocytes.

phosphatase score is reduced in about 90% of patients. There is an increase in the serum vitamin B_{12} concentration and the serum vitamin B_{12} binding capacity, due to increased production of transcobalamin I, a B_{12}-carrying protein released by granulocytes and their precursors.

The bone marrow is extremely hypercellular. There is hyperplasia of the neutrophil, eosinophil and basophil granulocyte series and an increase in megakaryocytes. In the chronic phase of the disease, less than 15% of nucleated marrow cells are blast cells. Trephine biopsies may show some increase in reticulin.

Progression of changes in CGL

Detailed follow-up studies of the survivors of the atomic bomb explosions in Japan in 1945 have elucidated the pattern of progression of changes in CGL (Kamada & Uchino 1978). The appearance of the Ph^1 chromosome is probably the first manifestation of the disease. The earliest change in the peripheral blood is an increase of the leucocyte count above the upper limit of normal (11×10^9/litre). At the same time, basophilia, thrombocytosis and the low leucocyte alkaline phosphatase make their appearance. As the count rises to 20×10^9/litre, the percentage of neutrophil precursors in the peripheral blood rises above 5% of the total white-cell count and the increase in serum vitamin B_{12} becomes apparent. Splenomegaly is found when the count is in the region of 50×10^9/litre and shortly after that symptoms arise. It has been calculated that if all the leukaemic cells were derived from a single cell with a Ph^1 chromosome, then it would take about 6 years for the leucocyte count to reach about 100×10^9/litre. The leucocyte count in CGL increases with time and the rate of increase is exponential; that is, the number doubles at regular intervals, the actual interval in which doubling takes place varies between patients, and is often over 70 days. The increase in total leucocyte count is accompanied by an increase in the size of the spleen and by a fall in haemoglobin concentration.

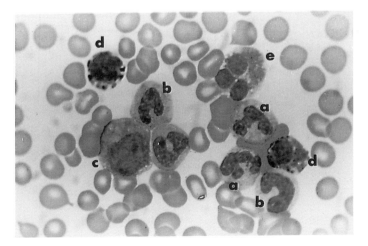

Fig. 7.8 Higher power view of some of the white cells from the blood film shown in Fig. 7.7. (a) Neutrophil granulocytes; (b) neutrophil metamyelocytes; (c) neutrophil myelocyte; (d) basophil granulocyte; and (e) eosinophil granulocyte.

Metamorphosis of CGL (acute-phase transformation)

All patients with chronic granulocytic leukaemia develop a more rapidly progressive terminal phase, although the exact form which this takes shows considerable variation between patients. The metamorphosis is the consequence of the evolution from the original Ph^1-positive clone of a new clone of leukaemic cells which is more malignant than the parent clone. The new clone, which may have additional chromosome abnormalities, either originates in an extramedullary site and subsequently spreads to the blood and marrow or originates in the bone marrow and spreads rapidly into the blood and other tissue. The cells which accumulate in acute-phase transformation are usually myeloblasts, but in a third of the patients they are lymphoblasts (blast cell transformation or blast crisis). Occasionally, they may be neutrophil promyelocytes, monoblasts, basophil or mast cell precursors, megakaryocytes or erythroblasts. The clinical features of transformation include fever, malaise, loss of weight, night sweats, bone pain, a rapidly enlarging spleen or extramedullary tumour mass, and resistance to standard therapy.

Treatment

Treatment is aimed at reducing the leucocyte count to normal limits, as experience has shown that this is followed by a marked alleviation of symptoms and rise in haemoglobin concentration.

A reduction in leucocyte count can usually be brought about by treatment with the alkylating agent, busulphan (Myleran). This drug may be administered continuously until the leucocyte count falls to about 20×10^9/litre. If the busulphan is then stopped, the leucocyte count will continue to fall for a few weeks and then start to rise. When the increase in cell count is relatively slow, busulphan can be given intermittently, recommencing therapy when the white-cell count rises to around 50×10^9/litre. However, if the white-cell count increases rapidly, a small maintenance dose may be given continuously. A clinical trial (Medical Research Council 1968) comparing busulphan therapy with intermittent radiotherapy to the spleen has shown that busulphan therapy is superior to radiotherapy. Busulphan may cause side effects such as pulmonary fibrosis, skin pigmentation and aplasia of the marrow. Hydroxyurea is a useful alternative to busulphan in the management of the chronic phase of CGL.

Irrespective of which cytotoxic drug is used, it is customary also to administer 300 mg allopurinol daily during the early phases of treatment to prevent marked increases in the uric acid level as a consequence of the destruction of tumour cells.

If symptoms related to hyperviscosity of the blood and leucocyte-related vascular obstruction are present in patients with very high white-cell counts, the counts should be rapidly reduced by repeated leucapheresis and high doses of hydroxyurea.

The median survival of patients with CGL who are treated with current cytotoxic drugs is 3–4 years, which is only slightly better than the median survival in untreated patients. Some patients survive for as long as 10–15 years. Once metamorphosis occurs, the outlook is bad; the majority of patients die within 1–2 months.

One form of treatment for patients under the age of 50 who have an HLA-compatible sibling is bone marrow transplantation in the chronic phase. Although this represents the only chance of cure, the procedure carries a substantial morbidity and mortality.

OBJECTIVES IN LEARNING

1   To know the more common causes of reductions and increases in the absolute counts of various types of white cell in the blood.

2   To be familiar with the aetiology, pathogenesis, clinical and haematological features and method of diagnosis of glandular fever.

3   To understand the classification of leukaemia into acute lymphoblastic, acute myeloid, chronic lymphocytic and chronic granulocytic based on the clinical picture and the cytological findings and to be aware of further schemes for subclassifying the acute leukaemias.

4   To know the causes of the symptoms and clinical features in leukaemia.

5   To know the natural history of the main types of leukaemia and the effects of treatment on it.

6   To know the basic principles (but not the details) of treatment in (a) acute leukaemia; (b) chronic granulocytic leukaemia; and (c) chronic lymphocytic leukaemia.

REFERENCES

Banatvala J.E. (1970) Infectious mononucleosis. Recent developments. (Annotation.) *Br. J. Haematol.*, **19**: 129.

Beeson P.B., Bass D.A. (1977) *The Eosinophil*. W.B. Saunders, Philadelphia.

Bennett J.M., Catovsky D., Daniel M.T., Flandrin G., Galton D.A.G., Gralnick H.R., Sultan C. (1976) Proposals for the classification of the acute leukaemias. *Br. J. Haematol.*, **33**: 451.

Bennett J.M., Catovsky D., Daniel M.T., Flandrin G., Galton D.A.G., Gralnick H.R., Sultan C. (1980) A variant form of hypergranular promyelocytic leukaemia (M3). *Br. J. Haematol.*, **44**: 169.

Bennett J.M., Catovsky D., Daniel M.T., Flandrin G., Galton D.A.G., Gralnick H.R., Sultan C. (1982) Proposals for the classification of the myelodysplastic syndromes. *Br. J. Haematol*, **51**: 189.

Butturini A., Gale R.P. (1989) Annotation: chemotherapy versus transplantation in acute leukaemia. *Br. J. Haematol.*, **72**: 1.

Carter R.L. (1966) Review of some recent observations on 'glandular fever cells'. *J. Clin. Pathol.*, **19**: 448.

Dameshek W. (1967) Chronic lymphocytic leukeamia—an accumulative disease of immunologically incompetent lymphocytes. *Blood*, **29**: 566.

Editorial (1983) The hypereosinophilic syndrome. *Lancet*, **i**: 1417.

Hamblin T.J., Oscier D.G. (1987) The myelodysplastic syndrome—a practical guide. *Hematol Oncol.* **5**: 19–34.

Kamada N., Uchino H. (1978) Chronological sequence of appearance of clinical and laboratory findings characteristic of chronic myelocytic leukemia. *Blood*, **51**: 843.

Maldonado J.E., Hanlon D.G. (1965) Monocytosis: a current appraisal. *Mayo Clin. Proc.*, **40**: 248.

Medical Research Council (1968) Chronic granulocytic leukaemia. Comparison of radiotherapy and busulphan therapy. Report of MRC working party for therapeutic trials in leukaemia. *Br. Med. J.*, **1**: 201.

Pullen H. (1973) Infectious mononucleosis. *Br. Med. J.*, **2**: 350.

Rai K.R., Sawitsky A., Cronkite E.P., Chanana A.D., Levy R.N., Pasternak B.S. (1975) Clinical staging of chronic lymphocytic leukemia. *Blood*, **46**: 219.

RECOMMENDED READING

Catovsky D. (ed.) (1981) *The Leukaemic cell*. Churchill Livingstone, Edinburgh.

Galton D.A.G. (1982) The chronic leukaemias. In: *Blood and its Disorders* (eds. R.M. Hardisty and D.J. Weatherall), 2nd edn, pp. 877–917. Blackwell Scientific Publications, Oxford.

Mahmoud A.A.F., Austen K.F., Simon A.S. (1980) *The Eosinophil in Health and Disease*. Grune & Stratton, New York.

Chapter 8
Chronic Myeloproliferative Disorders

The chronic myeloproliferative disorders are a group of related conditions characterized by the proliferation of a neoplastic clone of low malignancy derived from a pluripotent or multipotent haemopoietic stem cell. The four conditions which are included under this heading are polycythaemia rubra vera; essential thrombocythaemia; idiopathic myelofibrosis and chronic granulocytic leukaemia. Some authors exclude chronic granulocytic leukaemia from this group but there is no valid reason for doing so, there being no fundamental difference between the chronic phase of chronic granulocytic leukaemia and the three other conditions. Although many patients with a chronic myeloproliferative disorder can be classified into the four conditions at diagnosis, there are a number of unclassifiable patients with intermediate characteristics who clearly belong with this group. Except in idiopathic myelofibrosis, the abnormal clone generates increased concentrations of one or more of the following cell types in the peripheral blood: erythrocytes, platelets, granulocytes and monocytes. Some patients with polycythaemia rubra vera and essential thrombocythaemia and occasional patients with chronic granulocytic leukaemia develop extensive myelofibrosis during the course of their illness. The fibroblasts responsible for the myelofibrosis in these conditions as well as in idiopathic myelofibrosis do not belong to the neoplastic clone; the fibrosis seems to result from the release of fibroblast-stimulating factors by abnormal megakaryocytes (i.e. the fibrosis is reactive). Another common feature of the chronic myeloproliferative disorders is that they may all terminate in acute leukaemia. Treatment of these disorders is usually aimed not at cure but at alleviating symptoms and reducing the risk of serious complications; however, some patients with chronic granulocytic leukaemia may be cured by marrow transplantation (p. 129).

The myelodysplastic syndromes resemble the chronic myeloproliferative disorders in resulting from the proliferation of an abnormal clone of low malignancy derived from a haemopoietic stem cell. The distinction between the two types of disease is based on the finding of disordered maturation of blood cells (dysplasia) at presentation in the former but not the latter.

Since a progressive and marked increase in the leucocyte count is the most striking haematological feature of chronic granulocytic leukaemia, this disorder is discussed in the section on leukaemia on p. 125 rather than in this chapter.

POLYCYTHAEMIA RUBRA VERA (primary proliferative polycythaemia)

Polycythaemia rubra vera is a chronic disease in which there is a slowly expanding mutant cell clone derived from a multipotent haemopoietic stem cell. The mutant clone gives rise to increased numbers of red cells and, often, also of neutrophils and platelets. The erythroid progenitor cells (p. 2) derived from the clone are abnormal in that they form colonies *in vitro* in the absence of added erythropoietin. The clonal nature of the abnormal cell population has been shown by the demonstration that in women with polycythaemia vera who are heterozygous at the X-chromosome-linked locus for glucose-6-phosphate dehydrogenase, the red cells, granulocytes and platelets contain only one of the two isoenzyme types, whereas cells unaffected by the disease (e.g. skin fibroblasts) contain both. Most of the symptoms and complications of the disease can be attributed to the high red-cell count and packed cell-volume (PCV) which causes an increase in blood volume and viscosity. The latter leads to a decreased blood flow through the tissues.

Clinical features

Patients are usually aged between 40 and 70 years. In the early stages of the disease there may be no symptoms and a raised haemoglobin concentration may be an incidental finding. Symptoms are often insidious in onset and numerous. They include headache, dizziness, tinnitus, a feeling of fullness in the head, weakness, insomnia, visual disturbances, generalised pruritus, dyspnoea on exertion, angina and claudication. Some patients present acutely with a thrombotic or haemorrhagic episode (Calabresi & Meyer 1959; Videbaek 1975; Berlin 1975, 1976).

Venous thromboses and superficial thrombophlebitis are more common than arterial thromboses. There may be thrombosis of deep veins (sometimes with embolism), or of mesenteric, splenic, portal or hepatic veins. Arterial thromboses may cause cerebral or cardiac infarcts or peripheral gangrene (Fig. 8.1). In Videbaek's series from Copenhagen (1950), nearly one-third of the patients had thrombotic episodes and these accounted for 20% of the deaths. The incidence of vascular occlusion has been found to be correlated directly with the PCV (Pearson & Wetherley-Mein 1978). Patients with a PCV greater than 0.6 have occlusive episodes at a rate of almost one each year (Fig. 8.2). The risk of vascular occlusion is also greater in patients with high platelet counts than in those with normal counts.

Some patients have peptic ulcers and may bleed from them, but there is uncertainty as to whether the incidence of peptic ulceration is greater than in the normal population. About 10% of cases suffer from gout secondary to increased haemopoietic activity and the consequent increase in nucleic acid turnover and uric acid production.

Haemorrhagic manifestations may also occur and include ecchymoses, epistaxis and life-threatening intra- and post-operative bleeding. The cause of the bleeding is not well-understood. It may be related to the presence of abnormally large platelets with functional defects (e.g. diminished response to aggregating agents such as ADP, see p. 165).

On examination, there may be a florid dusky-red colour of the face, lips, hands and feet, congestion of the conjunctival vessels and marked distension of retinal veins. Splenomegaly, usually of moderate degree, is seen in about 70% of patients at presentation. The liver is enlarged in half the cases.

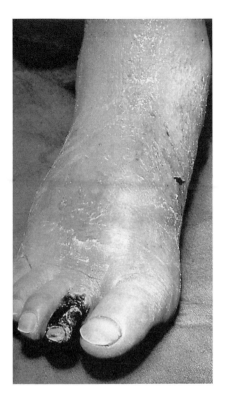

Fig. 8.1   Gangrene of a toe in a patient with polycythaemia rubra vera.

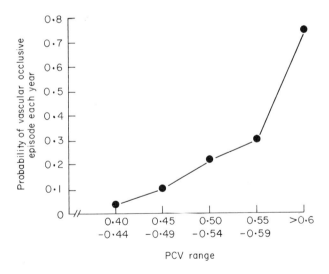

Fig. 8.2   The probability of the occurrence of a vascular occlusive episode related to the PCV. A probability of 0.1 indicates a 1 in 10 chance of the occurrence (adapted from Pearson & Wetherley-Mein 1978).

Laboratory findings

The haemoglobin concentration, red-cell count and PCV are high; haemoglobin values of 18–24 g/dl are common and the PCV is usually well over 0.47 in females and 0.52 in males. The total red-cell volume (measured using ^{51}Cr-labelled red cells) is increased, indicating the presence of true polycythaemia. The total plasma volume (measured using ^{125}I-labelled albumin) is usually decreased or normal and the total blood volume is increased. The red cells are usually normochromic and normocytic. However they may be hypochromic and microcytic due to absolute or relative iron deficiency. A true iron deficiency may result from recurrent spontaneous gastrointestinal haemorrhage and repeated venesection. A relative iron deficiency arises from the inability of a normal store of body iron to meet the needs of a markedly expanded red cell renewal system. Other haematological features are:

1 a neutrophil leucocytosis (usually up to 30×10^9/litre) in 75% of cases, often with some metamyelocytes and myelocytes on the blood film;
2 a raised or normal neutrophil leucocyte alkaline phosphatase score;
3 an increase in the absolute basophil count in some cases;
4 a raised platelet count (up to 1000×10^9/litre or higher) in two-thirds of the cases;
5 an elevated serum vitamin B_{12} level due to an increase in transcobalamin I;
6 increased whole blood viscosity;
7 decreased plasma and urinary erythropoietin levels;
8 hyperuricaemia in 70% of patients.

In most cases, marrow smears and trephine biopsies show an increase in cellularity, with a corresponding reduction in fat cells. The increased cellularity is caused by hyperplasia particularly of the erythropoietic cells but also of the granulocytopoietic cells and megakaryocytes.

Differential diagnosis

Other causes of true polycythaemia (i.e. causes of secondary polycythaemia, see p. 21) must be excluded by appropriate investigations (e.g. intravenous pyelography to exclude renal lesions). A definite diagnosis of polycythaemia rubra vera may be made when an increase in red-cell mass is associated with either splenomegaly or at least two of the following: neutrophil leucocytosis; thrombocytosis; high neutrophil alkaline phosphatase score and elevated serum vitamin B_{12} level. When the increased red-cell mass is not associated with these diagnostic features (and secondary polycythaemia has been excluded), the condition is best described as idiopathic erythrocytosis. On prolonged follow-up, some patients with idiopathic erythrocytosis eventually develop the full-blown picture of polycythaemia rubra vera, but others do not.

Treatment and prognosis

The aim of treatment is to maintain the PCV below 0.50, and preferably below 0.45, and thus prevent dangerous thrombotic episodes (see Fig. 8.2). Venesection relieves symptoms rapidly and is the treatment of choice in the first instance. If long-term control of the PCV requires frequent venesections (e.g. more than

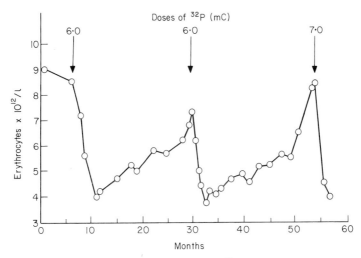

Fig. 8.3   The effect of giving three doses of ^{32}P on the erythrocyte count of a patient with polycythaemia vera (adapted from Szur *et al.* 1959).

once every 2 months) or if there is a substantial thrombocytosis (venesection may actually increase the thrombocytosis), continuous or intermittent treatment with busulphan or hydroxyurea, or irradiation of the bone marrow using an intravenous injection of radioactive phosphorus (^{32}P) (Szur *et al.* 1959) should be instituted. A single injection of ^{32}P often controls both the high PCV and high platelet count for more than 1 year. Further injections may be given when necessary (Fig. 8.3).

The survival from diagnosis is 18 months in untreated patients and 8–16 years in patients adequately treated with venesection alone, venesection plus an alkylating agent or venesection plus ^{32}P. The clinicopathological picture of idiopathic myelofibrosis develops in 30% of cases and of acute leukaemia in about 10%. The incidence of terminal acute leukaemia is higher in patients treated with busulphan or ^{32}P than in those treated with venesection alone.

ESSENTIAL THROMBOCYTHAEMIA

This chronic myeloproliferative disorder is usually seen in middle aged or elderly individuals and is closely related to polycythaemia rubra vera. It is characterized by:

1   recurrent bleeding due to abnormal platelet function (e.g. gastrointestinal haemorrhage, haematuria and bruising);

2   episodes of both arterial and venous thrombosis;

3   a very high platelet count (usually in the range 1000×10^9/litre to 4000×10^9/litre);

4   some abnormally large platelets with bizarre shapes;

5   a hypercellular bone marrow with a marked increase in the number of megakaryocytes (Silverstein 1968; Frick 1969). Megakaryocytes are larger than normal. Glucose-6-phosphate dehydrogenase isoenzyme studies have shown

Table 8.1   Causes of thrombocytosis.

Reactive
Haemorrhage, haemolysis, trauma, surgery,
    post-partum, recovery from thrombocytopenia
Acute and chronic infections
Chronic inflammatory disease (e.g. ulcerative colitis,
    rheumatoid arthritis)
Malignant disease (e.g. carcinoma, Hodgkin's disease)
Splenectomy and splenic atrophy
Iron deficiency anaemia

Chronic myeloproliferative disorders
Essential thrombocythaemia, polycythaemia rubra vera, chronic
    granulocytic leukaemia, idiopathic myelofibrosis

that the platelets are derived from a single mutant cell clone. There is often a moderate neutrophil leucocytosis and a basophilia. The haemoglobin concentration is either normal or slightly increased. Iron deficiency anaemia due to chronic gastrointestinal blood loss may develop and the serum uric acid level may be raised. Thrombotic episodes are seen more frequently in older patients and are presumably caused by a combination of the very high platelet count and degenerative vascular disease. The spleen is enlarged early in the disease but eventually undergoes atrophy from repeated infarction. The disease runs a chronic course and evolves into myelofibrosis in 8% of cases and into acute leukaemia in about 10%.

The differential diagnosis includes other chronic myeloproliferative disorders and a reactive thrombocytosis (Table 8.1).

Busulphan, melphalan or ^{32}P are effective in reducing the platelet count to below 500×10^9/litre and so preventing thrombotic and haemorrhagic complications. Symptoms such as intermittent digital ischaemia and transient cerebral ischaemic attacks may respond to inhibitors of platelet aggregation such as aspirin and dipyridamole; however, since platelet function is abnormal in this condition, these drugs could increase the risk of haemorrhage.

IDIOPATHIC MYELOFIBROSIS (MYELOSCLEROSIS, AGNOGENIC MYELOID METAPLASIA)

Studies using glucose-6-phosphate dehydrogenase isoenzyme markers and cytogenetic markers have confirmed the presence of a neoplastic clone derived from a multipotent haemopoietic stem cell in idiopathic myelofibrosis. The fibroblasts found in the bone marrow are not part of the abnormal clone. It is thought that the neoplastic clone generates abnormal megakaryocytes which release fibroblast-stimulating factors and thereby cause fibrosis of the marrow.

Idiopathic myelofibrosis is a chronic disorder usually found between the ages of 40 and 70 years. Its main features are:

1   moderate to gross splenomegaly (Fig. 8.4), sometimes causing abdominal discomfort;

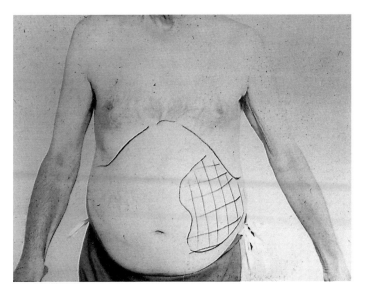

Fig. 8.4 Gross splenomegaly in a patient with idiopathic myelofibrosis.

2 constitutional symptoms such as anorexia, weight loss, fever and night sweats (usually in the later stages of the disease);

3 a leucoerythroblastic anaemia (p. 109);

4 the presence of many tear-drop-shaped poikilocytes in the blood film (Plate 29);

5 progressive fibrosis of the marrow and, in some cases, a thickening of the bone trabeculae (osteosclerosis);

6 extramedullary haemopoiesis (Videbaek 1975).

The white cell and platelet counts may be increased early in the disease but are reduced later. The neutrophil alkaline phosphatase score is frequently raised but may be normal or even low. Red cells may show a defect similar to that seen in paroxysmal nocturnal haemoglobinuria (p. 51) and occasional patients have haemoglobinuria. Hyperuricaemia may cause gout. X-rays of the axial skeleton show increased bone density (due to osteosclerosis) in about half of the patients.

Marrow aspiration is often unsuccessful and the diagnosis is made by performing a trephine biopsy of the marrow (Figs. 8.5, 8.6). During the early phases of the disease there is hypercellularity of all cell lines in the marrow, including megakaryocytes, and minimal fibrosis. Eventually, there is a marked reduction of haemopoietic tissue associated with a gross increase in reticulin fibres. There is also an increase in collagen fibres and fibroblasts. A number of diseases such as carcinomatosis, Hodgkin's disease and tuberculosis are sometimes associated with extensive fibrosis of the marrow (Bain & Wickramasinghe 1986) and such causes of secondary myelofibrosis must be excluded (Fig. 8.7).

No treatment is usually given until fairly late in the course of the disease. Markedly anaemic patients require regular blood transfusion. Folic acid, 5 mg

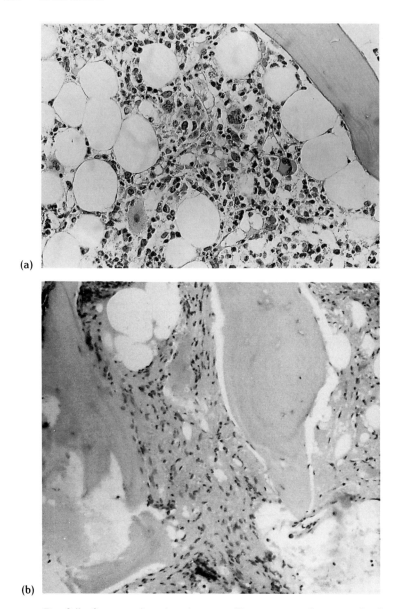

(a)

(b)

Fig. 8.5 Sections of trephine biopsies of bone marrow (haematoxylin & eosin). (a) Specimen from haematologically normal individual. (b) Specimen from a patient with idiopathic myelofibrosis showing replacement of some of the haemopoietic cells by fibroblasts and collagen.

daily, is often prescribed as the increased proliferative activity in the marrow increases folate requirements and may cause folate deficiency. Busulphan (carefully administered in low dosage) or hydroxyurea may be effective in reducing the size of a large spleen that is causing substantial discomfort; allopurinol should be given simultaneously to prevent urate nephropathy and

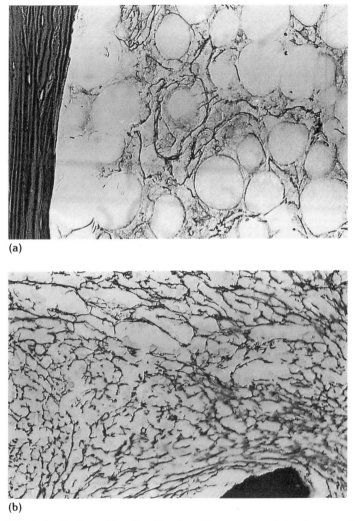

Fig. 8.6 Sections of trephine biopsies of bone marrow (silver impregnation of reticulin). (a) Specimen from haematologically normal individual. (b) Specimen from a patient with idiopathic myelofibrosis showing an increase in the quantity of reticulin fibres.

gout. Splenectomy may decrease excessive transfusion requirements or improve troublesome thrombocytopenia when these are related to pooling of cells within the spleen and to hypersplenism. However, there is a significant mortality from haemorrhage and infection during the post-operative period.

The median survival from diagnosis is 4–5 years. However, survival for 10–20 years is reasonably common. Patients die from bleeding, cardiac failure, infection and thrombosis. Acute leukaemia develops terminally in 10–20% of cases.

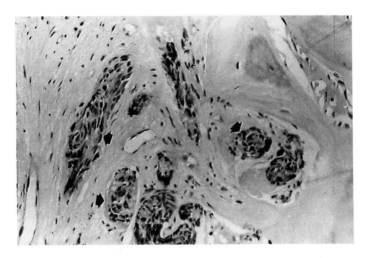

Fig. 8.7 Trephine biopsy of bone marrow showing metastases from a carcinoma (arrows) and fibrosis of the surrounding marrow (i.e. secondary myelofibrosis).

OBJECTIVES IN LEARNING

1 To know the features common to this group of disorders.

2 To know the pathogenesis, clinical and laboratory manifestations and the natural history of the four main chronic myeloproliferative disorders and current approaches to therapy.

3 To understand the differential diagnosis of polycythaemia, a high platelet count and myelofibrosis.

REFERENCES

Bain B.J., Wickramasinghe S.N. (1986) Pathology of the marrow: general considerations. In: *Blood and Bone Marrow, Systemic Pathology* (ed. S.N. Wickramasinghe) (3rd edn), Vol 2, p. 73. Churchill Livingstone, Edinburgh.

Berlin N.I. (ed.) (1975, 1976) Polycythaemia I & II, *Semin. Hematol.* vol. 12.4 & 13.1 Grune & Stratton, New York.

Calabresi P., Meyer O.O. (1959) Polycythaemia vera. I. Clinical and laboratory manifestations. *Ann. Int. Med.*, **50**: 1182.

Frick P.G. (1969) Primary thrombocythemia. *Helv. Med. Acta*, **35**: 20.

Pearson T.C. & Wetherley-Mein G. (1978) Vascular occlusive episodes and venous hematocrit in primary proliferative polycythaemia. *Lancet*, **ii**: 1219.

Silverstein M.N. (1968) Primary or haemorrhagic thrombocythemia. *Arch. Intern. Med.*, **122**: 18.

Szur, L., Lewis S.M., Goulden A.W.G. (1959) Polycythaemia vera and its treatment with radioactive phosphorus. *Quart J. Med.*, **28**: 397.

Videbaek A. (1950) Polycythaemia vera. Course and prognosis. *Acta Med. Scand.* **138**: 179.

Videbaek A. (ed.) (1975) Polycythaemia and myelofibrosis. *Clin. Haematol.*, vol. 4.2. W.B. Saunders, Philadelphia.

Chapter 9
Aplastic Anaemia and
Pure Red Cell Aplasia

ACQUIRED APLASTIC AND HYPOPLASTIC ANAEMIA

Acquired aplastic anaemia is a disorder characterized by a pancytopenia, i.e. a reduction in the number of red cells, neutrophils and platelets in the peripheral blood, and a decrease in the amount of haemopoietic tissue in the bone marrow. No other evidence of a disease process affecting the marrow, such as leukaemia, myeloma or carcinoma is present. It is an uncommon disease, the prevalence in Europe being between 1 and 3 per 100 000 people.

Aetiology

In about half the cases, no aetiological factors can be identified and such cases are described as having idiopathic acquired aplastic anaemia. In the others, the aplasia is associated with exposure to certain drugs or chemicals, ionizing radiation, or certain viruses.

Most cases of secondary aplastic anaemia result from an idiosyncratic reaction to the use of antirheumatic drugs (e.g. phenylbutazone, oxyphenbutazone, indomethacin, propionic acid derivatives such as ibuprofen, or sodium aurothiomalate), chloramphenicol or trimethoprim-sulphamethoxazole (co-trimoxazole). Many other drugs have been less commonly implicated and these include anticonvulsants (phenytoin, troxidone), anti-diabetic drugs (chlorpropamide and tolbutamide), mepacrine, organic arsenicals and potassium perchlorate. Benzene is the only industrial chemical which often produces aplastic anaemia if inhaled in sufficient dose; trinitrotoluene, certain insecticides, carbon tetrachloride, and glues can also cause aplasia of the marrow.

Aplastic anaemia may develop after a single massive dose of whole-body irradiation (e.g. during atomic bomb explosions or radiation accidents). It was also seen in the past following repeated radiotherapy to the spine in patients with ankylosing spondylitis.

Severe aplastic anaemia, usually with a poor prognosis, may rarely develop in children and young adults about 10 weeks after a hepatitis A or non-A, non-B infection. Marrow aplasia is also a rare complication of Epstein–Barr virus infection.

The T-lymphocytes of some patients with acquired aplastic anaemia inhibit the *in vitro* growth of haemopoietic colonies from autologous and allogeneic bone marrow. This finding, together with the response of about 50% of patients to antilymphocyte globulin, raises the possibility that autoimmune mechanisms may be involved in the aetiology of the aplasia in a number of cases.

Pathogenesis

It is generally considered that the pancytopenia and marrow aplasia are largely the consequence of damage to the multipotent haemopoietic stem cells. This damage results in a marked depression in the rate at which the stem cells differentiate into committed haemopoietic progenitor cells.

Clinical features

Both idiopathic and secondary aplastic anaemia occur at all ages. The onset is often insidious but may be acute. Symptoms include:

1   lassitude, weakness and shortness of breath due to the anaemia;
2   haemorrhagic manifestations resulting from the thrombocytopenia;
3   fever and recurrent infections as a consequence of the neutropenia.

Haemorrhagic manifestations include epistaxis, bleeding from the gums, menorrhagia, bleeding into the gastrointestinal and urinary tracts and ecchymoses and petechiae. The severity of the symptoms is variable and depends on the severity of the cytopenias. In patients with severe neutropenia and thrombocytopenia, fulminating infections (e.g. pneumonia) and cerebral haemorrhage are common causes of death. In secondary aplastic anaemia, symptoms may appear several weeks or months, or occasionally, one or more years after discontinuation of exposure to the causative drug or chemical. Splenomegaly is rare in aplastic anaemia, and if the spleen is palpable alternative diagnoses should be explored.

Haematological findings

There is a normochromic or macrocytic anaemia, usually associated with a low reticulocyte count. The platelet count is invariably below 100×10^9/litre and may be much lower. A neutropenia and monocytopenia are usually found at some stage of the disease. Some patients also have a reduced absolute lymphocyte count. There is a marked increase in serum and urinary erythropoietin levels.

Markedly hypocellular marrow fragments are usually found in marrow smears, most of the volume of the marrow fragments being made up of fat cells (Plate 7). Haemopoietic cells of all types, including megakaryocytes, are decreased or absent, and in severe aplastic anaemia the majority of the cells seen are plasma cells, lymphocytes and macrophages. Residual erythropoietic cells are morphologically abnormal. Although the marrow is generally hypocellular, it contains some foci of normal or even increased cellularity. Thus, even in patients with severe aplastic anaemia, marrow aspiration may occasionally yield normocellular or hypercellular fragments. In order to obtain a reliable estimate of marrow cellularity, it is essential to examine histological sections of a trephine biopsy of the iliac crest. This not only provides a larger volume of marrow for study than a single marrow aspirate but also permits the detection of foci of leukaemia cells, myeloma cells or carcinoma cells, if present.

Some patients with acquired aplastic anaemia develop the red cell defect seen in paroxysmal nocturnal haemoglobinuria (p. 51), without or with haemoglobinuria. Occasional patients develop a terminal acute leukaemia.

Diagnosis

Other causes of pancytopenia (particularly, aleukaemic leukaemia) should be considered and excluded before a diagnosis of aplastic anaemia is made. The causes of pancytopenia are summarized in Table 9.1.

Prognosis

Patients with both idiopathic and secondary acquired aplastic anaemia show a highly variable clinical course. About 15% of patients have a severe illness from the outset and die within 3 months of diagnosis. Overall, as many as 50% of cases die within 15 months of diagnosis and 70% within 5 years. Only about 10% make a complete haematological recovery. If a patient survives for longer than 18 months, there is a reasonable chance of prolonged survival and complete recovery. Poor prognostic features include a platelet count less than 20×10^9/litre, a neutrophil count below 0.2×10^9/litre, a reticulocyte count under 10×10^9/litre and marked hypocellularity of the marrow.

Treatment

If a causative drug or chemical is identified, exposure to this agent should be immediately stopped. Supportive therapy including red cell transfusions and antibiotics should be administered when necessary; the extent of supportive therapy required depends on the degree of cytopenia. Platelet transfusions are only indicated if haemorrhage becomes a serious problem, as repeated platelet transfusions lead to alloimmunization and a reduction of the efficacy of subsequent platelet transfusions. If marrow transplantation is planned, the administration of blood products should be limited to the bare minimum, since multiple transfusions have an adverse effect on the outcome of transplantation.

Bone marrow transplantation is indicated at diagnosis for patients under 40 years with severe aplastic anaemia (i.e. showing the poor prognostic features mentioned above), particularly if an HLA-compatible sibling donor is available. Patients who are not transplanted may benefit from treatment with antithymocyte globulin, androgens or the anabolic steroid oxymetholone (which causes less virilization of females than androgens).

Table 9.1   Causes of pancytopenia.

Mainly due to a failure of production of cells
Bone marrow infiltration: leukaemia
    (including aleukaemic leukaemia, p. 120), myeloma, carcinoma (Plate 30),
    myelofibrosis, lipid storage disorders, marble bone disease
Severe vitamin B_{12} or folate deficiency
Aplastic or hypoplastic anaemia

Mainly due to an increased peripheral destruction of cells
Splenomegaly
Overwhelming infection
Systemic lupus erythematosus
Paroxysmal nocturnal haemoglobinuria (p. 51)*

---

*In some cases, there is also an impaired production of cells due to hypoplasia of the marrow

Table 9.2   Causes of pure red cell aplasia.

Congenital
Diamond–Blackfan syndrome (congenital erythroblastopenia or
    erythrogenesis imperfecta)

Acquired
Idiopathic
Viral infections:
    Parvovirus B19 (p. 29)
Other viral infections: primary atypical pneumonia, infectious mononucleosis, mumps
Drugs and chemicals:
    Benzene, phenytoin sodium, azathioprine
Thymic tumours
Other malignant diseases:
    Hodgkin's disease, carcinoma
Automimmune disorders:
    SLE, rheumatoid arthritis
Renal insufficiency
Protein-energy malnutrition

CONGENITAL PANCYTOPENIA (familial hypoplastic anaemia, Fanconi syndrome)

The features of this rare disorder are:

1   inheritance as an autosomal recessive character;

2   onset of pancytopenia between the ages of 5 and 10 years;

3   frequent association with other congenital abnormalities (e.g. skin pigmentation, short stature, microcephaly, skeletal defects, genital hypoplasia and renal abnormalities);

4   various chromosomal abnormalities (e.g. chromatid breaks) in haemopoietic cells, lymphocytes and skin fibroblasts;

5   increased incidence of acute leukaemia and solid tumours.

There is usually some response to treatment with androgens and corticosteroids.

PURE RED CELL APLASIA

Rarely, aplasia or severe hypoplasia affects only the erythropoietic cells. Patients with this abnormality have anaemia and reticulocytopenia together with normal white cell and platelet counts. Pure red cell aplasia may present as an acute self-limiting condition (e.g. when it follows a parvovirus infection) or as a chronic disorder. The causes of pure red cell aplasia are listed in Table 9.2. Immunological mechanisms may underlie the aplasia in some patients (e.g. those with thymoma or autoimmune disorders). The diagnosis of pure red cell aplasia may be followed by the development of acute myeloid leukaemia several years later.

OBJECTIVES IN LEARNING

1   To know the aetiology of acquired aplastic anaemia, including the drugs that have been most commonly reported to cause this syndrome.

2 To know the clinical and laboratory features, the natural history, and the principles of treatment of acquired aplastic anaemia.

3 To understand the difference between aplastic anaemia and pure red cell aplasia.

RECOMMENDED READING

Beard M.E.J. (1976) Fanconi anaemia. In: *Ciba Foundation Symposium 37 (new series) on Congenital Disorders of Erythropoiesis* (eds. R. Porter and D.W. Fitzsimons), pp. 103–114. Elsevier, Amsterdam.

Buckner C.D., *et al.* (1982) Bone marrow transplantation, in *Recent Advances in Haematology 3* (ed. A.V. Hoffbrand). Churchill Livingstone, Edinburgh.

Camitta B.M., Storb R., Thomas E.D. (1982) Aplastic anaemia. *N. Eng. J. Med.*, **306**; 645 and 712.

Geary C.G. (ed.) (1979) *Aplastic Anaemia*. Ballière Tindall, London.

Gordon-Smith E.C. (1983) Management of aplastic anaemia. *Br. J. Haematol.* **53**; 185.

Krantz S.B. (1973) Pure red cell aplasia. *Br. J. Haematol.* **25**; 1.

Thomas E.D. (ed.) (1978) Aplastic Anaemia. *Clinics in Haematology*, vol 7.3, W.B. Saunders, Philadelphia.

Williams D.M., Lynch R.E., Cartwright G.E. (1973) Drug induced aplastic anemia. *Semin. Hematol.* **10**: 195.

Chapter 10
Myeloma, other Paraproteinaemias and Lymphoma

MULTIPLE MYELOMA

Multiple myeloma is a disease arising from the malignant transformation of a B-cell or, possibly, a pre-B or earlier cell (Barlogie *et al* 1989). The differentiating cells of the malignant clone have the morphology of plasma cells or plasmacytoid lymphocytes and usually secrete a monoclonal immunoglobulin (Ig), a monoclonal light chain, or both. Such monoclonal proteins are called paraproteins; they consist of structurally identical molecules and, therefore, produce a discrete band (M band) on electrophoresis. The primary site of proliferation of the malignant cells is the bone marrow which shows many nodules of tumour tissue as well as diffuse interstitial infiltration (Fig. 10.1). Osteoclasts are stimulated by a factor secreted by the myeloma cells and this together with the expansion of the intramedullary tumour cell mass leads to multiple well-defined osteolytic lesions, generalized osteoporosis and hypercalcaemia. Marrow infiltration also causes impairment of haemopoiesis and haematological abnormalities. Some patients with IgA paraproteins (which tend to polymerize) and a few patients with high levels of IgG3 paraproteins have a substantially raised plasma viscosity and may suffer from the hyperviscosity syndrome (p. 147). Light chains are filtered through the glomeruli and are found in the urine; they may eventually damage the renal tubules. In 10% of patients, the paraprotein is converted into deposits of amyloid in various tissues. Levels of normal immunoglobulins are reduced and in advanced disease there is a

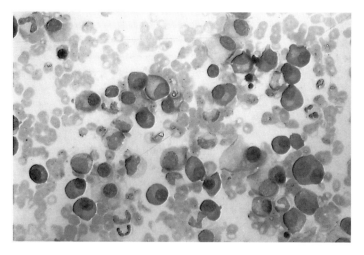

Fig. 10.1 Bone marrow smear from a patient with multiple myeloma showing infiltration by myeloma cells. There are only a few normal haemopoietic cells.

reduction in circulating T-cells. Extramedullary tumour deposits develop frequently.

Clinical features

The incidence of myeloma is 3–6 per 100 000 of the population per year. Most patients are between the ages of 50 and 70 years. There is a prolonged asymptomatic phase which may last for a number of years. The most common presenting symptom is bone pain usually over the lumbar spine. Pathological fractures are frequent and often affect the lower thoracic and upper lumbar vertebrae and the ribs. Compression fractures of the vertebrae may damage the spinal cord or spinal roots and cause neurological symptoms. Large tumours may form in relation to any bone and cause pressure symptoms.

Renal failure may be found at presentation or develop during the course of the disease. Chronic renal failure commonly results from obstruction of renal tubules by proteinaceous casts leading to tubular atrophy and interstitial fibrosis (myeloma kidney). Renal dysfunction may also result from the toxic effects of light chains on tubule cells, the deposition of light chains in glomeruli and amyloidosis. Acute renal failure may be precipitated by dehydration, hypercalcaemia or hyperuricaemia.

Other features of myelomatosis include:

1 symptoms of anaemia (p. 16);

2 recurrent bacterial infections due mainly to decreased levels of normal immunoglobulin but also to neutropenia;

3 systemic symptoms of hypercalcaemia such as anorexia, vomiting, lethargy, stupor or coma;

4 peripheral and autonomic neuropathy, macroglossia, cardiomegaly, diarrhoea and carpal tunnel syndrome due to amyloidosis.

Peripheral neuropathy may also be caused by infiltration of nerves by plasma cells or by a direct toxic effect of the paraprotein. The hyperviscosity syndrome may occasionally develop. This is characterized by neurological disturbances (dizziness, somnolence and coma), cardiac failure and haemorrhagic manifestations. Spontaneous haemorrhages may also occur in the absence of hyperviscosity due to an adverse effect of the paraprotein on coagulation and platelet function and, in the later stages of the disease, due to thrombocytopenia. A few paraproteins are cryoglobulins and may cause symptoms such as urticaria and acrocyanosis, when the patient becomes cold.

Laboratory findings

A normochromic normocytic anaemia is common. When the disease is advanced, thrombocytopenia and neutropenia may also be found. The blood film may show a leucoerythroblastic picture and occasional plasma cells; red cells may show an increased tendency to form rouleaux and the paraprotein may cause an increased basophilic staining of the background in between red cells. The ESR is often raised, sometimes to more than 100 mm/hour. The serum uric acid is raised in about half the cases (and may contribute to the renal damage).

Bone marrow aspirates usually contain a greatly increased proportion of plasma cells (Plates 31, 32). The latter may either appear normal or show various atypical features such as marked pleomorphism, pronounced multinuclearity, immaturity of the nucleus (i.e. finely distributed chromatin and nucleoli) and dissociation between nuclear and cytoplasmic maturation. Some aspirates may show only a slight increase in plasma cells (5–10% of nucleated marrow cells as compared with 0.1–2% in normal marrow) and others may show no increase. The latter results from the multifocal nature of the plasma cell infiltrate.

Electrophoresis of serum usually demonstrates the monoclonal Ig as a discrete band (M-band) and the nature of the paraprotein can be determined by immunoelectrophoresis. Each Ig class may be quantitated using radial immunodiffusion. Light chains (also called Bence–Jones proteins) cannot usually be detected in the serum except when there is impairment of renal function. They are present in urine and are best detected and studied by electrophoresis and immunoelectrophoresis of concentrated urine. Conversely, whole immunoglobulin molecules only appear in the urine when there is renal damage. In 50% of patients with myeloma, the paraprotein is IgG, in 25% it is IgA, in 20% it is light chain only and in 1–2% it is IgD or IgE. IgM-producing myelomas are extremely rare. Over half the patients with an IgG- or IgA-secreting myeloma have monoclonal light chains in their urine; in two-thirds of these patients the light chain is k and in the remainder it is λ. In 1–2% of patients with myeloma, paraprotein cannot be detected in either serum or concentrated urine (nonsecretory myeloma).

Diagnosis

This is often based on the finding of at least two of the following three features:
1   a monoclonal Ig in the serum or monoclonal light chains in the urine or both;
2   an increased proportion of plasma cells (often with atypical features) in marrow aspirates;
3   discrete osteolytic lesions on X-ray studies (Fig. 10.2).
The differential diagnosis is from a benign paraproteinaemia (p. 150).

Treatment

Cytotoxic drug therapy is usually reserved for symptomatic patients and patients with any renal dysfunction (Galton 1981). Melphalan or cyclophosphamide is given either intermittently or, in smaller doses, continuously. Most patients respond, with an improvement in symptoms, a rise in haemoglobin and a gradual reduction in the paraprotein levels. Treatment reduces the tumour mass and is usually stopped when the paraprotein level stops falling. Combination chemotherapy may be more effective in younger patients and is also given to patients who fail to respond to single drug therapy.

Prognosis

The median survival from diagnosis is 2–3 years. Asymptomatic patients with a Hb >10 g/dl and blood urea $\leq$8 mmol/l have a 75% chance of surviving 2 years. By contrast, patients who are restricted in their activity and who have either a Hb $\leq$7.5 g/dl or a blood urea > 10 mmol/l have only a 10% chance of surviving 2 years. Patients eventually become refractory to chemotherapy and die of renal failure or infection. A few patients develop a myelodysplastic syndrome or terminal acute myeloid leukaemia or immunoblastic lymphoma.

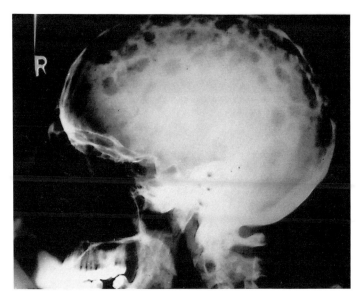

Fig. 10.2 Radiograph of the skull of a patient with multiple myeloma showing multiple discrete radiolucent lesions with no sclerosis at the margin.

Solitary plasmacytoma

Solitary tumours consisting of malignant plasma cells may be found in the bone marrow or in extramedullary sites such as the upper respiratory tract. It is usual to find a monoclonal immunoglobulin in the serum or monoclonal light chains in the urine, or both. In the case of extramedullary plasmacytomas, there is often no evidence of tumour elsewhere and the prognosis after excision followed by local radiotherapy is very good.

OTHER PARAPROTEINAEMIAS

Waldenström's macroglobulinaemia

In this condition, there is a malignant monoclonal proliferation of a cell belonging to the B-lineage. The incidence is about 10% of that of multiple myeloma. The tumour cells are found in peripheral lymphoid tissue, bone marrow and other tissues and, in some patients, also in the peripheral blood. They have the morphology of plasmacytoid lymphocytes and secrete an IgM paraprotein and thus differ from myeloma cells which very rarely secrete this class of paraprotein. Symptoms result both from tissue infiltration and from hyperviscosity of the blood caused by the paraprotein. Unlike in multiple myeloma, osteolytic lesions are rare.

Heavy chain diseases

In these rare paraproteinaemias, the B-lineage-derived malignant clone secretes γ, α or μ heavy chains rather than complete immunoglobulin molecules. The clinical picture is that of a lymphoma; α-chain disease is characterized by severe malabsorption due to infiltration of the small intestine by lymphoma cells.

Other lymphoproliferative disorders

A paraprotein may also be found in chronic cold haemagglutinin disease (p. 50), and in some patients with malignant lymphoma or chronic lymphocytic leukaemia.

Benign paraproteinaemia (benign monoclonal gammopathy or monoclonal gammopathy of uncertain significance, MGUS)

A paraprotein is found in the serum in 0.1–1.0% of normal adults and in 3% of subjects over 70 years. A high proportion of such individuals suffer from a condition termed benign paraproteinaemia that does not require treatment; in this condition, the abnormal clone, derived from the B-cell lineage, behaves like a benign neoplasm. Benign paraproteinaemia is characterized by:

1   the absence of osteolytic lesions;
2   the presence of relatively low levels of serum paraprotein (<20 g/l) which remain stable over a long period of follow-up;
3   the absence of light chains or the presence of very low concentrations (<500 mg/day) of light chains in the urine;
4   normal levels of immunoglobulins of classes other than the paraprotein class;
5   the finding of less than 5–10% of plasma cells in the bone marrow (i.e. only a slight plasmacytosis in the marrow);
6   the absence of marrow failure.

MALIGNANT LYMPHOMAS

The malignant lymphomas are tumours of peripheral lymphoid tissue in which the transformed cell is either a cell belonging to the lymphocyte series or a histiocyte. The expansion of the malignant cell clone causes a partial or complete loss of normal lymph node architecture and a progressive enlargement of lymph nodes. Although the bone marrow and peripheral blood may contain lymphoma cells at some stage, the predominant pathological manifestations are in extramedullary tissue (usually, lymph nodes). The malignant lymphomas are subdivided into Hodgkin's disease and the non-Hodgkin's lymphomas.

Hodgkin's disease

In this condition the affected lymph nodes (Fig. 10.3) are infiltrated by abnormal mononucleate cells, large binucleate cells called Reed–Sternberg cells, lymphocytes, plasma cells, macrophages, eosinophils and fibrous tissue. The Reed–Sternberg cells and their mononuclear counterparts possess vesicular nuclei with prominent eosinophilic nucleoli. They are thought to be the malignant cells and to be derived from dendritic reticulum cells. The other cell types infiltrating the lymph nodes are probably normal cells that are reacting against the tumour cells.

Clinical features

The age-related incidence curves are bimodal with one peak in young adults and the other in old age. The male: female ratio is about 2:1, but the nodular

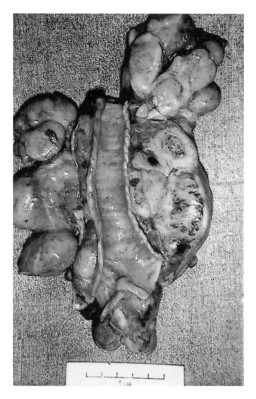

Fig. 10.3 Post-mortem findings in a patient with advanced Hodgkin's disease. The mediastinal glands are greatly enlarged due to infiltration by tumour tissue.

sclerosing type of the disease (p. 153) is predominantly seen in young females. The disease has an insidious onset. The most common presentation is gradual enlargement of one group of lymph nodes. The disease then spreads to adjacent lymph node areas via the lymphatics and eventually metastasizes via the blood to extranodal sites. The cervical lymph nodes are affected first in 56% of cases and the mediastinal, axillary, abdominal and inguinal glands in 15, 11, 4 and 9%, respectively. The enlarged glands vary in size from 1 to 8 cm in diameter and are usually discrete, painless and rubbery. Splenomegaly may be present (Fig. 10.4). Hepatomegaly and involvement of other extra-nodal tissue is usually seen late in the course of the disease; the affected tissues include the skin, stomach, small intestine, bone, lung and central nervous sytem.

Systemic symptoms are frequently present and may sometimes precede the detection of lymphadenopathy. Such symptoms include fever, pruritus, weight loss, lassitude, night sweats. Sometimes the fever is cyclic with several days of high swinging fever alternating with afebrile periods (Pel–Ebstein fever).

Haematological features
There is usually a normochromic normocytic anaemia and a high ESR. A neutrophil leucocytosis is seen in 30% of patients and eosinophilia in 15–20%.

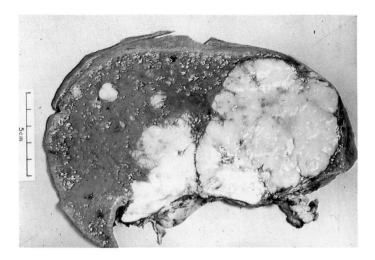

Fig. 10.4   Enlarged spleen from a patient with Hodgkin's disease. About half the cut surface of the spleen is occupied by masses of pale lymphoma tissue.

Marrow infiltration may occur and lead to a leucoerythroblastic blood picture. Lymphopenia due to a reduction in T-lymphocytes occurs late in the disease and is associated with an impairment of cell-mediated immunity and a consequent susceptibility to certain viral, fungal and protozoal infections and tuberculosis.

Histopathology of lymph nodes

There is complete or partial loss of the normal architecture due to infiltration by malignant and inflammatory cells. The diagnosis is based on finding Reed–Sternberg cells in the appropriate cellular background of mononuclear Hodgkin's cells, lymphocytes, neutrophil polymorphs, eosinophils and plasma cells (Kaplan 1980). Four different histopathological appearances are encountered in Hodgkin's disease and these are described in Table 10.1.

Staging and treatment

The extent of dissemination of malignant cells at presentation influences both the prognosis and the choice of therapy. Clinical staging involves not only a full clinical examination but also various investigations including chest X-ray, trephine biopsy of the bone marrow, and CT scanning of the abdomen. Table 10.2 summarizes the features of the Ann Arbor staging system which is commonly used to assess the spread of the disease. Each stage is subdivided into A or B depending on whether systemic symptoms are absent or present, respectively. If a staging laparotomy with splenectomy, a wedge-biopsy of the liver and abdominal lymph node biopsy are performed, about one-third of cases initially considered to be in stages I or II are found to also have subdiaphragmatic disease and have to be placed in stages III or IV. However, most clinicians do not regularly perform staging laparotomies in such cases as the improved accuracy

Table 10.1 Rye classification of the histological appearances of lymph nodes in Hodgkin's disease.

Subgroup	Characteristics	Cases (%)	Surviving 5 years (%)
Lymphocyte predominance	Infiltrate consists largely of small lymphocytes. There are only a few eosinophils, Reed–Sternberg cells and mononuclear Hodgkin's cells	15	70
Nodular sclerosing	The node is divided by broad bands of connective tissue into nodules containing a mixture of Reed–Sternberg cells, mononuclear Hodgkin's cells, lymphocytes, plasma cells, macrophages and eosinophils	40	60
Mixed cellularity	There are no broad bands of connective tissue. The node is diffusely infiltrated with the same mixture of cell types as above. Reed–Sternberg cells are readily seen. Fibrosis and focal necrosis are common	30	30
Lymphocyte depletion	Mononuclear Hodgkin's cells and Reed–Sternberg cells are present in large numbers. Relatively few lymphocytes are seen and there may be diffuse fibrosis	15	20

in staging achieved in this way is not reflected in improved survival. This is mainly because patients who relapse after radiotherapy respond well to chemotherapy.

Megavoltage radiotherapy is the treatment of choice for stages I and IIA, cyclical combination chemotherapy or radiotherapy for stage IIB and cyclical combination chemotherapy for stages III and IV and for patients who relapse

Table 10.2 Basic features of the Ann Arbor staging system.

Stage	Characteristics
I	Involvement of one lymph node area
II	Involvement of two or more lymph node areas on the same side of the diaphragm
III	Involvement of lymph nodes on both sides of the diaphragm with or without involvement of the spleen
IV	Involvement of one or more extranodal sites (e.g. liver, marrow, lung)

after radiotherapy. Chemotherapy is sometimes also used as first line therapy for stage IIA with involvement of three or more nodal sites. Radiotherapy may beused following chemotherapy for the treatment of bulky or painful nodal or extranodal tumour masses and ulcerating skin lesions. The most commonly used drug combination is leukeran (chlorambucil), vincristine (Oncovin), procarbazine and prednisolone (LOPP).

Prognosis

This is related to both the histological type and clinical staging. Radiotherapy cures (10-year disease-free survival) over 90% of patients in stage I and over 80% in stage II. Combination chemotherapy induces a complete remission in 80% of cases in stages IIIB and IV and a 5-year disease-free survival in 50%.

Non-Hodgkin's lymphoma

A number of biologically distinct tumours arising from cells of lymphoid tissue are included in this category. About 75% of non-Hodgkin's lymphomas (including all follicular lymphomas) arise from cells of the B-cell lineage and most of the remainder from those of the T-cell lineage. The non-Hodgkin's lymphomas are currently classified into a number of types largely on the basis of the histological and cytological features of the tumour tissue (Canellos 1979; Lennert 1981; Wright 1982). On the basis of clinicopathological correlations, these various types are assigned one of two or three grades of malignancy (low-grade and high-grade, or low-grade, intermediate-grade and high-grade).

Aetiology

The aetiology is unknown. Patients with certain inherited or acquired immune deficiency syndromes (e.g. sex-linked agammaglobulinaemia, AIDS, patients with renal and heart transplants receiving immunosuppressive therapy) have an increased incidence of non-Hodgkin's lymphoma, as do survivors of the atomic bomb explosions in Japan. The African type of Burkitt's lymphoma is associated with malaria, EB virus infection (Bird & Britton 1982) and one of three specific chromosome translocations which result in the activation of an oncogene, *myc* (p. 116). In most cases of follicular lymphoma, a chromosomal translocation, t(14;18), juxtaposes the *bcl-2* oncogene on chromosome 18 next to the heavy chain locus on chromosome 14.

Clinical features

Painless enlargement of lymph nodes is the most frequent complaint. In general, the extent of spread of the disease at presentation is greater than in Hodgkin's disease. Hepatosplenomegaly is often found and other extranodal sites such as the bone marrow, nervous system, nasopharynx, gastrointestinal tract and skin are commonly involved. Constitutional symptoms are less frequent than in Hodgkin's disease and occur late in the course of the illness.

Haematological features

A normochromic normocytic anaemia is usually found and may be due to marrow infiltration, autoimmune haemolysis or splenomegaly and hypersplenism. Lymphoma cells may be present in the blood, with or without an associated lymphocytosis. In about 10% of patients there is an IgG or IgM paraprotein.

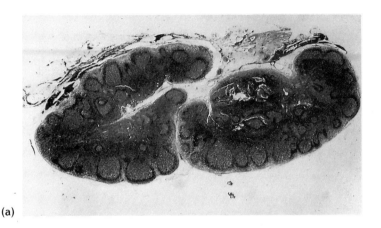

(a)

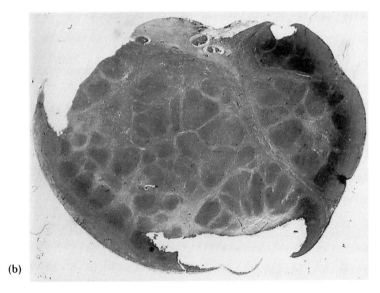

(b)

Fig. 10.5. (a) Section of antigen-stimulated human lymph node. The lymphoid follicles are confined to the cortex (B-cell area) and have an outer darkly-staining zone containing small lymphocytes and a pale germinal centre containing centroblasts (follicle centre cells), dendritic cells and macrophages. (b) Section of a lymph node infiltrated by a follicular (nodular) lymphoma. Note that the nodules of lymphoma cells are found throughout the lymph node, being present not only in the cortex but also in the paracortex (normally a T-cell area) and medulla (normally a follicle-free T- and B-cell area). (Courtesy of Dr R.D. Goldin.)

Fig. 10.6   Section of lymph node affected by a diffuse lymphoma. The diffuse infiltration by lymphoma cells has resulted in a complete loss of nodal architecture. (Courtesy of Dr R.D. Goldin.)

Histopathology of lymph nodes

Rappaport (1977) divided non-Hodgkin's lymphomas into nodular (follicular) or diffuse, depending on whether the tumour cells formed discrete nodules or diffusely infiltrated the lymph nodes (Figs. 10.5, 10.6). The tumours were then subclassified according to the cell types present into well- or poorly-differentiated lymphocytic lymphomas, histiocytic lymphomas, mixed lymphocytic and histiocytic lymphomas and undifferentiated lymphomas. This classification is being replaced by newer ones largely because surface marker studies of tumour cells have shown that in most tumours, cells described by Rappaport as histiocytes are in fact not histiocytes but lymphoid cells.

One of several schemes now used for the histopathological categorization of non-Hodgkin's lymphomas is the Kiel classification. This is based on the hypothesis that such tumours are derived from normal counterparts seen during the antigen-stimulated proliferation of B or T cells in peripheral lymphoid tissue and that the malignant cells retain morphological similarity with their putative normal counterparts, being unable to mature further. The cytological stages through which B cells progress following stimulation with specific antigen include centrocytes (which are small or large cells with cleaved nuclei), lymphoblasts (which are medium-sized cells with rounded nuclei and inconspicuous nucleoli), centroblasts (which are large cells with rounded nuclei and several peripheral nucleoli) and immunoblasts (which are very large cells with a rounded nucleus and, often, a single large central nucleolus). Both centrocytes and centroblasts are seen in normal germinal centres and the end-result of antigen-mediated stimulation of B cells is the formation of plasma cells or memory B cells. The features of the Kiel classification are given in Table 10.3.

Table 10.3   Kiel classification of non-Hodgkin's lymphoma.

Low-grade malignancy
Lymphocytic (B, T)
Lymphoplasmacytoid (B)
Centrocytic (B)
Centrocytic/centroblastic (B)

High-grade malignancy
Centroblastic (B)
Lymphoblastic (B,T)
   Burkitt type
   convoluted-cell type
   others
Immunoblastic (B,T)

True 'histiocytic'*
Malignant histiocytosis*

---

*Derived from cells of the mononuclearphagocyte system

Treatment and prognosis

The staging system described for Hodgkin's disease is used to determine the extent of dissemination at presentation; however, the clinical stage correlates less well with prognosis than in Hodgkin's disease. Patients with low-grade tumours are often in stage IV at presentation and an appreciable percentage of patients with high-grade tumours are in stages I or II.

Some asymptomatic patients with low-grade tumours in whom the disease progresses very slowly need not be treated at presentation. Symptomatic patients or patients with progressive disease may be treated with local radiotherapy if in stages I and II or with chemotherapy if in stages III and IV. Either single agent therapy with chlorambucil or combination chemotherapy with cyclophosphamide, vincristine (Oncovin) and prednisolone (COP) are effective. Although most patients with low-grade lymphomas are incurable, their median survival is relatively long, being about 7 years.

In patients with high-grade lymphomas, radiotherapy is used for stage I disease and combination chemotherapy for stages II–V. Radiotherapy cures many patients in stage I. Intensive chemotherapy induces complete remissions in about half the patients and cures in 20–30%. A variety of combinations of cytotoxic drugs are being used; one well-tried combination is cyclophosphamide, hydroxydaunorubicin, vincristine and prednisolone (CHOP).

Some varieties of non-Hodgkin's lymphoma

Burkitt's lymphoma is a B-lymphoblastic lymphoma with specific cytological and histological features. Affected African children commonly present with a jaw tumour and non-African patients with an abdominal tumour.

The Sezary syndrome and mycosis fungoides are cutaneous T-cell lymphomas. Sezary's syndrome is characterized by intensely itchy erythroderma, exfoliative dermatitis, lymphadenopathy, hepatosplenomegaly and the presence of some lymphoma cells with cerebriform nuclei (Sezary cells) in the peripheral blood. Mycosis fungoides is characterized by the formation of plaques and nodules of tumour cells in the skin (Fig. 10.7). In this condition, extracutaneous spread only occurs late in the course of the disease.

OBJECTIVES IN LEARNING

1 To understand the meaning of the term paraprotein and to know the various clinical situations in which a paraprotein may be found.

2 To have a moderately detailed knowledge of the pathology, clinical features and diagnosis of myelomatosis and to understand the principles of treatment of this disorder.

3 To understand the pathological and clinical features and the principles of treatment of Hodgkin's disease and the non-Hodgkin's lymphomas. Details of the various histological classifications of non-Hodgkin's lymphomas need not beknown.

REFERENCES

Barlogie, B., Epstein, J., Selvanayagam, P., Alexanian, R. (1989) Plasma cell myeloma—new biological insights and advances in therapy. *Blood* **73**: 865–879.

Bird A.G., Britton S (1982) The relationship between Epstein–Barr virus and lymphoma. *Seminars in Haematology*, Vol 19, p. 285. Grune & Stratton, New York

Canellos, G.P. (1979) (Ed) The non-Hodgkin's lymphomas. *Clinics in Haematology*, vol. **8.3**. W.B. Saunders, Philadelphia

Galton, D.A.G. (1981) Myelomatosis. In: *Postgraduate Haematology*, A.V. Hoffbrand &S.M. Lewis (Eds.). Heinemann, London

Kaplan, H.S. (1980) *Hodgkin's disease*, 2nd edn. Harvard University Press, Cambridge, Massachusetts

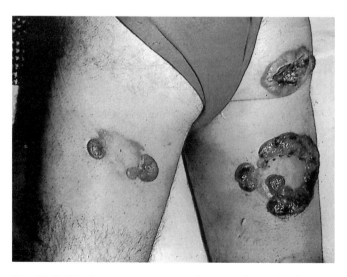

Fig. 10.7 Skin lesions in a patient with mycosis fungoides (a cutaneous T-cell lymphoma). The name of the disease is misleading; this condition is not caused by a fungus.

Lennert, K. (1981) *Malignant lymphomas other than Hodgkin's disease.* Springer Verlag, New York

Rappaport, H. (1977) Histological classification: non-Hodgkin's lymphoma. In: *Cancer Treatment Reports.* S.E. Janes & T. Grodden (Eds.). **61**: 1037–48

Wright, D.H. (1982) The identification and classification of non-Hodgkin's lymphoma: a review. *Diagnostic Histopathology* **5**: 73–111.

RECOMMENDED READING

Robb-Smith, A.H.T., Taylor, C.R. (1981) *Lymph node biopsy.* Miller Heyden, London

Salmon, S.E. (Ed)(1982) Myeloma and related disorders. *Clinics in Haematology,* vol. **11.1.** W.B. Saunders, Philadelphia

Stein, H., Gerdes J., Mason D.Y.(1982) The normal and malignant germinal centre. *Clinics in Haematology,* Vol **11.3**, pp. 531–560. W.B. Saunders, Philadelphia

Chapter 11
Haemostasis and Abnormal Bleeding

NORMAL HAEMOSTASIS

The cessation of bleeding following trauma to blood vessels results from three processes: (a) the contraction of vessel walls; (b) the formation of a platelet plug at the site of the break in the vessel wall; and (c) the formation of a fibrin clot. The clot forms within and around the platelet aggregates to form a firm haemostatic plug. The relative importance of these three processes probably varies according to the size of the vessels involved. Thus, in bleeding from a minor wound, the formation of a haemostatic plug is probably sufficient in itself, whereas, in larger vessels, contraction of the vessel walls also plays a part in haemostasis. The initial plug is formed almost entirely of platelets but this is too friable on its own and must be stabilized by fibrin formation.

CLASSIFICATION OF HAEMOSTATIC DEFECTS

Although the action of platelets, the clotting mechanism and the integrity of the vascular wall are all closely related in the prevention of bleeding, it is convenient to consider that abnormalities in haemostasis arise from defects in one of these three processes. The commonest cause of bleeding is undoubtedly a deficiency of platelets; the second commonest cause is an abnormality in the clotting mechanism. The remaining patients do not have any demonstrable lesion of the platelets or clotting mechanism and appear to be bleeding as a result of vascular abnormalities. The latter may be congenital as in hereditary haemorrhagic telangiectasia (Fig. 11.1) or acquired as in senile purpura, the Henoch-Schönlein syndrome (allergic purpura) and scurvy.

A clinical distinction can frequently be made between bleeding due to clotting defects and bleeding due to a diminished number of platelets. Patients with clotting defects usually present with abnormal bleeding in the deep tissues, that is, muscles or joints. On the other hand, patients with a deficiency of platelets usually present with superficial bleeding, that is, bleeding into the skin and from the epithelial surfaces of the nose, uterus and other organs. Haemorrhages into the skin occur in various sizes and include petechiae, which are less than 1 mm in diameter (Fig. 11.2) and ecchymoses, which are larger than petechiae and vary considerably in size (Fig. 11.3). A further useful clinical distinction is that bleeding usually persists from the time of injury in the case of platelet deficiency, since platelet numbers are inadequate to form a good platelet plug, whereas in clotting defects the initial bleeding may cease in the normal time since platelet plugs are readily formed, but as a consequence of the failure to form an adequate clot the platelet plug is not stabilized by fibrin formation and subsequently disintegrates, resulting in a delayed onset of prolonged bleeding. The clinical distinction is by no means complete, as deep-seated haemorrhage is sometimes

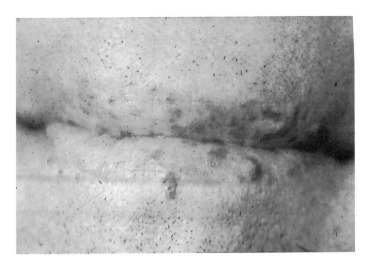

Fig. 11.1 Vascular malformations (reddish purple) on the lips of a patient with hereditary haemorrhagic telangiectasia; such lesions increase in number with advancing age. This rare condition is inherited as an autosomal dominant characteristic and may lead to recurrent gastrointestinal haemorrhage and chronic iron deficiency anaemia.

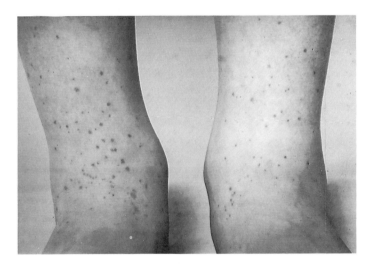

Fig. 11.2 Multiple pin-point haemorrhages (petechiae) on the legs of a patient with idiopathic autoimmune thrombocytopenic purpura.

found in platelet deficiency and, on the other hand, superficial bleeding may occur in clotting defects.

PLATELETS

Morphology and life-span

The blood platelets are formed in the bone marrow by the fragmentation of the cytoplasm of the megakaryocytes. They are discoid, non-nucleated (2–3 μm in

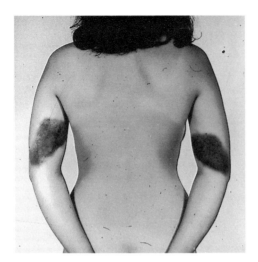

Fig. 11.3 Large ecchymoses on both upper arms of a woman with idiopathic autoimmune thrombocytopenic purpura.

diameter) and are normally present in a concentration of $160-450 \times 10^9$/litre of whole blood. Following their release from the marrow, their life-span is of the order of 10 days. This has been determined by labelling platelets with radioactive chromium (^{51}Cr). The shape of the survival curve obtained from radioactively labelled platelets is neither linear nor exponential and is difficult to interpret: it has been suggested that the platelets are delivered to the circulation with a potential life span of 9–12 days, but that there is also some random destruction irrespective of their age (Fig. 11.4). The sites of normal platelet destruction are not known.

Physiology

The main function of the platelets is the formation of the haemostatic plug, which incorporates several different physiological mechanisms (Mustard & Packham 1977). First there is the adherent property of platelets which enables them to stick to subendothelial collagen and microfibrils. Adhesion is brought about by the von Willebrand molecule (also known as Factor VIII Ag) present in the plasma and which has two receptor areas on its surface, one for the microfibrils and one for the platelet. Within 1–2 seconds after the platelets have become attached to exposed subendothelial structures, they change their shape from a disc to a more rounded form with spicules which encourage platelet–platelet interaction and they also release the contents of their granules, the most important substance released being adenosine diphosphate (ADP). The platelets are also stimulated to produce the prostaglandin, thromboxane A_2. The release of ADP and thromboxane A_2 causes an interaction of other platelets with the adherent platelets and with each other (secondary platelet aggregation), thus leading to the formation of a platelet plug. Receptors for fibrinogen are exposed on the surface of activated platelets and fibrinogen plays a role in linking platelets together to form aggregates.

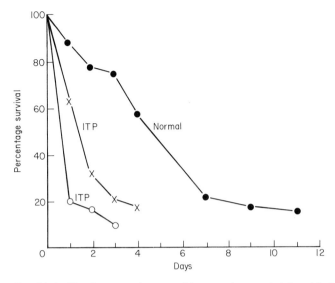

Fig. 11.4 Platelet survival curves: (•), normal survival; (x), mild idiopathic thrombocytopenic purpura; (○), severe idiopathic thrombocytopenic purpura. Adapted from Barkhan (1966).

Activation of Factor XII by contact with subendothelial structures initiates the formation of a fibrin clot around the platelet plug. When platelets aggregate, certain phospholipids (platelet factor 3) are exposed on their surface which promotes clotting by adsorbing other clotting factors and thus considerably enhancing the speed of the clotting reaction. Factors VIII and IX are adsorbed and potentiate factor Xa formation and then factors Xa and V are adsorbed and this results in a thousand-fold increase in the rate of conversion of prothrombin to thrombin. Platelets are also responsible for the contraction of the fibrin clot once it has been formed. Thus, the surface of a platelet is a site where fibrin formation can take place, leading to the development of the fully stabilized haemostatic plug.

Tests of platelet function

The bleeding time

The bleeding time test was introduced in 1911 by Duke, not as a diagnostic procedure, but as a means of following the progress of patients with thrombocytopenic purpura. When carried out under standardized conditions, it still remains the best clinical screening test that we have for the estimation of platelet function.

Bleeding time is estimated by making small wounds in the skin of the forearm after applying a blood-pressure cuff to the upper arm and inflating to 40 mm Hg; the average time that elapses until bleeding ceases is then measured. The wounds are three punctures made with a lancet in the method of Ivy or one or two short incisions in the various template methods; the depth of the wound is standardized. The normal range depends on the method and is 2–4 minutes with the Ivy method. Since the wound only damages small vessels, haemostasis is mainly dependent on the formation of a platelet plug and hence the bleeding time is prolonged when platelet numbers are reduced. It is almost always normal in the presence of clotting defects.

The bleeding time is dependent on both the number of platelets in the plasma and on the extent of their functional activity. When the functional activity is normal, then there is a good correlation between the platelet count and the bleeding time measured in minutes (Harker & Slichter 1972) (Fig. 11.5). Bleeding times are not prolonged until the platelet count has fallen to 100×10^9/litre. Below that value, there is a progressive and proportional prolongation in bleeding time, the time lengthening from the normal average of about 3 minutes to reach about 30 minutes as the platelet count falls to 10×10^9/litre. Below 10×10^9/litre, bleeding times may be prolonged to 1 hour or more.

On the other hand, when there are functional changes in platelet activity, bleeding times are either shorter or longer than might be expected from platelet numbers. For instance, in the autoimmune thrombocytopenias, almost all the platelets are younger than normal and are functionally more efficient. The bleeding times are thus shorter than might have been expected from platelet numbers (see Fig. 11.5). In contrast, there is a functional impairment of platelet activity in uraemia, in von Willebrand's disease and after the ingestion of aspirin, resulting in bleeding times that are prolonged despite platelet numbers in the normal range (see Fig. 11.5). Aspirin has a moderate effect on the bleeding time; 2 hours after the ingestion of 600 mg of aspirin, the bleeding time rises above the normal range in 30% of subjects and may be as long as 20 minutes. This prolongation is sufficient to provoke abnormal bleeding in certain people and aspirin is contraindicated in those with bleeding disorders. Aspirin acts by acetylating cyclo-oxygenase and this inhibits thromboxane A_2 synthesis with a subsequent reduction in platelet aggregation. The effect of a single dose of

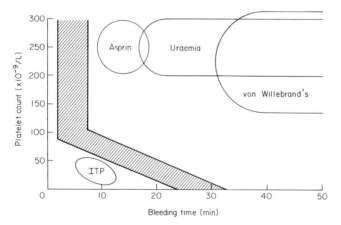

Fig. 11.5 The relationship between the platelet count and the bleeding time. The hatched area gives the relationship for platelets with normal functional activity. In idiopathic autoimmune thrombocytopenic purpura (ITP), the platelets are younger, larger and functionally more efficient. In uraemia, von Willebrand's disease and after taking aspirin, there is a functional impairment of platelet activity.

aspirin can be detected for 1 week, i.e. until most of the platelets present at the time of taking the aspirin have been replaced by newly formed platelets.

Estimation of the bleeding time is thus most useful when there are moderate to gross changes in the functional activity of the platelets. When the test is combined with an estimate of platelet numbers, it can differentiate between decreased and increased functional activity.

Other tests

A large number of *in vitro* tests of platelet function have been described. The most commonly used tests study the aggregation of platelets following the addition of adenosine diphosphate, adrenaline, thrombin, collagen and ristocetin to platelet-rich plasma. Aggregation causes a decrease in optical density and the test is performed using special equipment capable of continuously recording optical density.

RELATIONSHIP BETWEEN THROMBOCYTOPENIA AND ABNORMAL BLEEDING

It is well known that bleeding into the skin (petechial haemorrhages and ecchymoses) and bleeding from other sites may occur when the number of platelets falls below 100×10^9/litre. Gaydos et al. (1962) found a good inverse relationship between the platelet count and the number of days on which haemorrhage occurred if patients with leukaemia were analysed as a group (Fig. 11.6). At levels between 20 and 100×10^9/litre, petechiae, ecchymoses and nose bleeds were the commonest symptoms, but below 20×10^9/litre, gross haemorrhage (melaena, haematemesis, haematuria) become increasingly common. However, there is a great deal of variation in the relationship between the platelet count and haemorrhage in individual patients. Other factors clearly play a part in the control of haemostasis.

The reason for the occurrence of spontaneous haemorrhage when the platelet count is low is not known, but two possible mechanisms can be suggested. One, that the minor trauma associated with normal movement of the body causes capillary damage and that there is an insufficient number of platelets to form an adequate plug to prevent bleeding. The other suggested mechanism is that platelets continuously play a normal role in strengthening capillary walls by becoming attached and incorporated into endothelial cells. Although there is some evidence for the latter suggestion, it is by no means substantiated.

CAUSES OF THROMBOCYTOPENIA

Purpura is the collective term for bleeding into the skin or mucous membranes. The problem posed to the physician by a patient with purpura is a complex one, since the bleeding may result from a number of abnormalities in haemostasis and may be found associated with a large number of disease conditions. The solution of the problem must therefore be attempted in two stages.

1   Determination of the nature of the abnormality in the haemostatic process that results in bleeding; i.e. whether the defect is due to a low platelet count, a functional abnormality of the platelets, a deficiency of one or more clotting factors or a vascular defect.

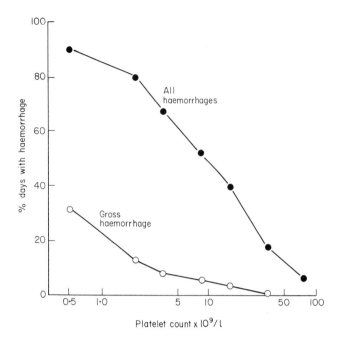

Fig. 11.6 Relationship between the platelet count and the number of days, expressed as a percentage, on which haemorrhage occurred in 92 patients with leukaemia. 'All haemorrhages' include petechiae, ecchymoses, epistaxis, haematuria, melaena and haematemesis. Note that gross haemorrhage only occurred when the platelet count fell below 20×10^9/litre. Adapted from Gaydos *et al.* (1962).

2 Correlation of this abnormality with others that may be present in order to obtain a diagnosis of the disease process (e.g. failure of platelet production by megakaryocytes due to marrow infiltration by leukaemic tissue). Patients presenting with purpura as a main sign can be separated into those with low platelet counts (thrombocytopenic) and those with normal platelet counts (non-thrombocytopenic). The non-thrombocytopenic group can be subdivided into those patients who have qualitative platelet defects and a larger group who have vascular abnormalities. The latter is a miscellaneous group and contains such diseases as Henoch-Schönlein purpura (allergic purpura), hereditary haemorrhagic telangiectasia, scurvy, purpura senilis and the purpura of infectious diseases and will not be discussed further.

Division into the thrombocytopenic and non-thrombocytopenic groups can be carried out by estimating the number of platelets in the peripheral blood. Patients with bleeding manifestations resulting from a deficiency of platelets have a platelet count below 100×10^9/litre. If the patient is found to have a low platelet count, the next step is to determine whether this is due to a failure of platelet production by the megakaryocytes, to a shortened life-span of the platelets, or to increased pooling of platelets in an enlarged spleen. The distinction between the first two of these possibilities can be made by assessing the number of megakaryocytes in a marrow aspirate.

FAILURE OF PLATELET PRODUCTION

If megakaryocytes are few or absent, it may be assumed that platelet production is at fault. The bone-marrow smears may also reveal other features which indicate the nature of the disease if evidence has not already been obtained from the peripheral blood. Thus, there may be a generalized aplasia of the bone-marrow (aplastic anaemia) or a selective decrease in megakaryocytes caused by certain drugs and viruses. Another cause of reduced platelet production is marked infiltration of the marrow by malignant cells (e.g. in leukaemia, lymphoma, myeloma and carcinoma) or by fibrous tissue. Reduced platelet production may also occur in patients with normal or increased numbers of megakaryocytes when there is ineffective megakaryocytopoiesis as in severe vitamin B_{12} or folate deficiency or in myelodysplastic syndromes.

SHORTENED PLATELET SURVIVAL

If the megakaryocytes in the marrow are numerous, then the thrombocytopenia is usually due to an excessive rate of removal of platelets from the peripheral circulation. In most cases the destruction results from autoantibodies attached to the platelet surface and the disease is termed autoimmune thrombocytopenic purpura. Occasionally it is due to intravascular platelet consumption due to: (a) disseminated intravascular coagulation; (b) interaction with damaged small blood vessels (microangiopathic thrombocytopenia) as in thrombotic thrombocytopenic purpura or the haemolytic uraemic syndrome; or (c) passage through a giant haemangioma.

Idiopathic autoimmune thrombocytopenic purpura

The occurrence of a disease which is characterized by petechiae (see Fig. 11.2), bruising (see Fig. 11.3) and spontaneous bleeding from mucous membranes was first described by Werlhof in 1735. The association of these characteristics with a deficiency of platelets was recognized nearly 100 years ago. No other abnormality or causative factor could be found and hence the disease was termed idiopathic. During 1949–54, Ackroyd showed that thrombocytopenia in patients taking the sedative sedormid is due to the formation of an antibody against a complex of sedormid and the platelet; his explanation of the phenomenon is that sedormid forms a very labile union with the surface of the platelet and that the antibody then combines with the sedormid-platelet complex and this leads to the destruction of the platelets (Ackroyd 1962). These findings led others to search for anti-platelet antibodies in idiopathic thrombocytopenia. It is now known that most patients with a clinical diagnosis of idiopathic thrombocytopenic purpura have autoantibodies in their plasma and on their own platelets which results in a shortened life-span due to premature destruction in the spleen. The original evidence for the existence of antibodies was obtained *in vivo* by Harrington *et al* (1951) who showed that the transfusion of plasma taken from these patients into normal volunteers would cause prolonged thrombocytopenia (Fig. 11.7). The causative factor in the plasma was later shown to be an IgG immunoglobulin. This explanation is also consistent with the observation that children born to mothers with idiopathic thrombocytopenic purpura also have thrombocytopenia

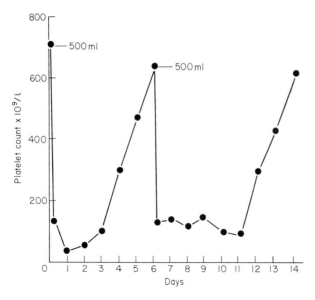

Fig. 11.7   The effect on the platelet count of a normal person of two transfusions of 500 ml of plasma from a patient with idiopathic thrombocytopenic purpura. The reduction in platelet count was due to the presence of anti-platelet antibodies in the donor's plasma. The high pre-treatment platelet count is due to the use of an indirect counting technique. Redrawn from Harrington (1951).

for the first few days of life, as would be expected since IgG antibodies are known to cross the placenta.

The platelet life-span has been shown to be shortened in all patients with immune thrombocytopenic purpura and is often reduced to about 1–2 days or less (e.g. 2 hours) compared to the normal life span of 10 days. Surface counting over the spleen and liver has shown that in approximately 30% of patients the destruction takes place only in the spleen, but that in the rest it also occurs in the liver.

Clinical features

Autoimmune thrombocytopenic purpura presents in both an acute and chronic form. The acute form is seen at all ages but is most common before the age of 10 years, and two-thirds of patients give a history of a common childhood viral infection (upper respiratory tract infection, rubella) preceding the purpura. Platelet counts are usually less than 50×10^9/litre. In most patients the disease runs a self-limiting course of 1 week to 6 months but in approximately 20% it becomes chronic, that is, lasts more than six months. The disease is almost always self-limiting when there is a history of preceding infection and in such cases may be caused by immune complexes rather than by platelet autoantibodies. The mortality is low, the main danger being intracranial bleeding.

The chronic form occurs mainly in the age period 10–30 years, although it is sometimes seen in older subjects; it has a higher incidence in women than in men. The chronic form is usually not severe and mortality is low; platelet counts are usually between 20 and 80 $\times$ 10^9/litre. Spontaneous cures are rare and the disease is characterized by relapses and remissions.

In a large series described by Doan et al (1960), about one-third of the patients without a history of preceding infection had petechiae and ecchymoses as the only presenting signs. The remainder also had bleeding from the following sites in order of frequency: nose, gums, vagina, gastrointestinal and renal tract. Cerebral haemorrhage occurred in 3%. As a general rule the spleen is not palpable; when it is palpable it usually, but not always, rules out the diagnosis.

Diagnosis

In order to make a diagnosis, bone marrow aspiration is often carried out. In idiopathic thrombocytopenia, megakaryocytes are increased in number (up to four- or eightfold) and in size. An absence or reduction of megakaryocytes rules out the idiopathic disease. The marrow aspiration also serves to exclude other causes of thrombocytopenia, such as aplastic anaemia, leukaemia or marrow infiltration by carcinoma cells, lymphoma cells or myeloma cells. Thrombocytopenia is sometimes the first sign of systemic lupus erythematosus. Thrombocytopenia due to drugs must also be excluded.

Treatment

In the acute form of the disease, over 80% recover whatever the form of treatment. Corticosteroids have been widely used, but there is evidence that they have no effect on the duration of thrombocytopenia and in one study appeared to delay recovery (Lusher & Zeulzer 1966). Nor is there any evidence that prednisone decreases the number of patients who proceed to the chronic form (Schulman 1964). On the other hand, steroids are very useful in the chronic forms of the disease, about 50% having a partial remission.

Splenectomy should be considered if the response to corticosteroids is poor or the dose of corticosteroid required to prevent bleeding is unacceptably high. Two-thirds of the patients will respond to this treatment, some permanently. However, some will relapse after an interval. It has been claimed that it is possible to predict the effect of splenectomy by determining the site of sequestration of ^{51}Cr-labelled platelets; splenectomy carried out when there was only splenic sequestration resulted in remission in 90% of patients, but when hepatic sequestration also took place it had little effect in 70% of the patients (Najean & Ardaillon 1971). However, others have found a good response to splenectomy even when destruction was mainly hepatic (Aster 1972).

Azathioprine or cyclophosphamide can be used in patients who fail to respond to splenectomy, in an attempt to reduce antibody formation. These drugs have been reported to be effective in some cases.

Recently, it has been found that large doses of intravenous gammaglobulin are a very useful form of therapy. Almost all patients with immune thrombocytopenia have an increase in platelet count lasting at least 2 weeks and some derive long-term benefit. Immunoglobulin probably acts by interfering with platelet destruction by inhibiting the binding of the Fc portion of the IgG antibodies on the platelet surface to Fc receptors on macrophages.

Secondary autoimmune thrombocytopenic purpura

An autoimmune thrombocytopenia may precede other manifestations of systemic lupus erythematosus (SLE) by several years and may complicate the course of SLE, other autoimmune disorders, lymphoma and chronic lymphocytic leukaemia. Patients infected with the human immunodeficiency virus (HIV) may develop immune thrombocytopenia long before developing other characteristic features.

Drug-induced immune thrombocytopenia

Certain drugs such as quinine, quinidine and allylisopropylcarbamide (Sedormid) cause a shortening of platelet life-span by one of two mechanisms. Firstly, the drug or a metabolite binds to a plasma protein, and antibodies form against and react with the drug-protein complexes. The resulting immune complexes react with platelets and cause their destruction ('innocent bystander' mechanism). Secondly, the drug or a metabolite binds to platelets and antibody formed against the drug–platelet complex combines with platelets that have reacted with the drug but not with normal platelets.

PLATELET TRANSFUSIONS

It is often possible to raise the platelet count temporarily by platelet transfusions. The main indication for platelet transfusion is severe haemorrhage due to thrombocytopenia when the cause is diminished platelet production. When thrombocytopenia results from excess destruction, as in the presence of platelet antibodies, the response to transfusion is poor. The platelets are transfused as platelet concentrates and should be given within 5 days of withdrawal from the donor. Platelet counts need only be maintained above 20×10^9/litre since severe haemorrhage is rare above this level (Serpick 1965; Editorial in *Br Med J* 1971).Transfusion may also be indicated in a patient with thrombocytopenia prior to surgery (p. 200).

NORMAL COAGULATION MECHANISM

The classical theory of blood clotting put forward in 1904 stated that four components were involved: thromboplastin, calcium, prothrombin and fibrinogen. Little further progress was made in this ill-understood subject until 1947, when Owren in Norway discovered another component, factor V. Up to 1950, most of the work on blood clotting was carried out on what is now known as the extrinsic system and laboratory studies usually used the tissue factor, thromboplastin, to initiate clotting. It was thought that the reason why whole blood clotted after being withdrawn into a syringe was that thromboplastin was released from platelets or blood cells. About 1950 MacFarlane and his colleagues (MacFarlane 1967) started to investigate clotting without the addition of any tissue factors. This work resulted in the discovery of new clotting factors and the assignation of Roman numerals for the recognized clotting factors. It also led to the cascade hypothesis of blood coagulation (MacFarlane 1964, 1969). This hypothesis proposed that each clotting factor is present in the plasma as a proenzyme and that the conversion of the proenzyme to an active enzyme occurs on interaction with the appropriate activated clotting factor. It was considered that such conversions took place in a sequential manner and that each step in the sequence of interactions served as an amplification mechanism. Subsequent work has shown that the development of enzyme activity in a proenzyme results from the splitting of one or more peptide bonds, which brings about a conformational change in the molecule and reveals the active enzyme site.

There are two pathways or systems present within the cascade. First, there is the *intrinsic system*, all the components of which are in the plasma. The sequence of action of factors in the intrinsic system is XII, XI, IX (with VIII as cofactor), X, II and I, as illustrated in Figure 11.8. The clotting sequence is initiated by the adsorption of factor XII to exposed collagen and microfibrils which results in the appearance of an active enzyme site on the molecule (factor XIIa). This reaction is potentiated by two plasma proteins, prekallikrein (which becomes converted to kallikrein by factor XII) and high molecular weight kininogen. Factor XIIa then acts on XI to form the active enzyme XIa. Factor XI can also become activated by a different mechanism, namely adsorption to activated platelets in the platelet plug. This is clearly an important mechanism as people with a deficiency of factor XII do not have a significant bleeding tendency. Factor XIa then acts on IX to form IXa which then acts on X to form Xa, using factor VIII as a cofactor. Factor Xa then acts on factor II (prothrombin), using factor V as a cofactor to form factor IIa (thrombin). Factor IIa splits several small negatively charged peptide fragments from factor I (fibrinogen), thus removing repulsive forces from the molecule and allowing the remainder to polymerize and form the fibrin fibre. Finally, factor XIII, also present in the plasma,

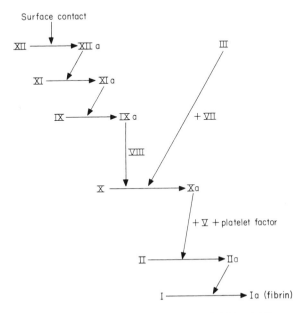

Fig. 11.8 Modification of MacFarlane's (1964, 1969) enzyme-cascade hypothesis regarding the sequence of reactions from surface contact to fibrin formation. The suffix 'a' denotes the enzymatically active form of each coagulation factor.

stabilizes and strengthens the fibrin polymers by forming covalent bonds between the fibrin chains (glutamine–lysine bridges).

The interaction of factors IX, VIII and X takes place mainly on the surface of platelets, where the rate of reaction is very considerably increased when compared to the rate occurring in solution. Hence bleeding in thrombocytopenia results from a failure of the clotting cascade as well as the lack of a platelet plug.

The amplification factor at each stage is not known, but if it were tenfold, then each molecule of factor XII activated by contact with a foreign surface would result in about one million molecules of fibrin.

Secondly, there is the *extrinsic system* which consists of two factors: factor III (also known as thromboplastin) which is released from damaged tissue, and factor VII, present in the serum as an inactive serine esterase. Following trauma, factors III and VII form a complex, factor VII becomes activated and then acts on X to form Xa. Both systems thus share a final common path (factor X, II and I). Calcium is required at several stages throughout the system.

Six of the synonyms for the factors are still in general use and should be known. They are: anti-haemophilic globulin, VIII; Christmas factor, IX; pro-thrombin, II; thrombin, IIa; fibrinogen, I; and fibrin, Ia.

Inhibitors of coagulation

Apart from the basic reactions mentioned above, there are additional interactions between various components of the coagulation mechanism, mainly in the form of positive and negative feedback systems. Thus, factors activated late in the sequence potentiate reactions at earlier stages (for instance, factor IIa potentiates the activity of factors VIII and V). There are also inhibitors which prevent localised fibrin formation from becoming widespread. The most important of these inhibitors are antithrombin III, protein C and protein S.

Antithrombin III

As its name implies, this is mainly an inhibitor of thrombin, but it also inhibits other factors earlier in the pathway; its action is markedly potentiated by heparin (Beresford 1988). Congenital antithrombin III deficiency is usually inherited as an autosomal dominant character; estimates of its prevalence have varied widely from 1 in 2 000 to 1 in 40 000. Heterozygotes may suffer from recurrent deep venous thrombosis, superficial thrombophlebitis and pulmonary embolism; the first thrombotic event usually occurs after the age of 15 years.

Protein C and protein S

Two other inhibitors of coagulation are the vitamin K-dependent substances protein C and protein S (Manucci & Tripodi 1988). Protein C becomes activated when it reacts with thrombin bound to thrombomodulin, a protein of the endothelial cell membrane. Activated protein C is a serine protease and inactivates factors V and VIII; it also promotes fibrinolysis. Protein S potentiates the effects of activated protein C.

Some individuals have a hereditary deficiency of protein C, with about 50% of normal levels; these are heterozygotes for a mutation affecting the protein C gene and are found with a prevalence of about 1 in 20 000. A proportion of such heterozygotes displays the clinical picture seen in inherited antithrombin III deficiency but in addition is particularly prone to develop superficial thrombophlebitis and cerebral vein thrombosis. Homozygotes for the mutant gene are rare and those who have virtually no protein C present with purpura fulminans or extensive thrombosis of visceral veins in the neonatal period.

The prevalence of hereditary protein S deficiency is about 1 in 20 000 and a proportion of heterozygotes for this defect suffers from recurrent venous thromboembolism. Interestingly, homozygotes are not much more severely affected than heterozygotes.

The incidence of protein C deficiency in children and adults below the age of 45 years with recurrent venous thrombosis is about 5–8% and the incidence of protein S deficiency in this group is similar.

THE FIBRINOLYTIC MECHANISM

The complex mechanism for producing fibrin is counterbalanced by a mechanism for the enzymatic lysis of clots. In order to explain the physiological role of the fibrinolytic system, it has been suggested, though not established, that fibrin is slowly but continuously deposited on the vascular endothelium in order to seal off any deficiencies that may occur, and that the purpose of the fibrinolytic system is to remove the fibrin once it has served its function.

The dissolution of the fibrin into fibrin-degradation products (FDP) is carried out by the proteolytic plasma enzyme plasmin. Plasmin is present in the plasma in an inactive form (plasminogen) and must be converted into the active form by tissue plasminogen activator, which is present in all tissues and is especially concentrated around blood vessels. Plasmin is not specific for fibrin but will also break down other protein components of plasma, including fibrinogen and the clotting factors V and VIII, and thus a mechanism is present which confines the activities of plasmin to fibrin (Fig. 11.9). The precise nature of this mechanism is still not clear, but it is thought that either plasminogen or the plasminogen activator or both are specifically adsorbed onto fibrin; plasmin is then formed from the plasminogen and digests the fibrin to which it is adsorbed. Under normal conditions, any plasmin released from the fibrin into the circulation is immediately inactivated by combining with the plasma inhibitor, α_2-antiplasmin. In this way, generalized breakdown of fibrinogen and other proteins does not occur.

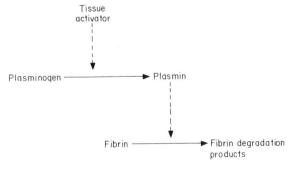

Fig. 11.9 The fibrinolytic mechanism. The continuous lines indicate conversion, the broken lines activity.

As well as tissue activator, physiological activators of plasminogen are present in many body secretions, especially in urine (urokinase) and in the pleural and peritoneal cavities. A single-chain form of urokinase and recombinant plasminogen activator injected intravenously or into the coronary artery are useful therapeutic agents for the treatment of early acute myocardial infarction. These drugs may also be useful in other types of thrombosis. Non-physiological activators, such as streptokinase, derived from certain streptococci, and acylated plasminogen–streptokinase activator complex (Apsac) are also being used as thrombolytic agents.

TESTS FOR CLOTTING DEFECTS

Once the sequence of events in clotting is understood, the tests for defects become simple to understand. There are only two basic tests which are widely used:

1   the *activated partial thromboplastin time* (e.g. kaolin–cephalin clotting time) which estimates the activity of the intrinsic system;
2   the *prothrombin time* which estimates the activity of the extrinsic system.

Clotting defects conveniently fall into two groups; in the first, and by far the largest, group are those patients with acquired deficiencies of several factors (II, VII, IX and X) resulting from treatment with coumarin drugs, vitamin K deficiency and liver disease. It can be seen from Fig. 11.8 that three of these factors lie in the extrinsic system and the specific test for the extrinsic system is the prothrombin time. In the second and much smaller group are those patients with congenital defects of one of the clotting factors. There are several recognized congenital clotting defects, but 80–90% of the patients in this group are haemophiliacs (factor VIII deficiency). About 10–20% have factor IX deficiency, and only about 1% have deficiencies of one of the other eight factors. Thus in practice almost all the congenital deficiencies involve factors in the initial stages of the intrinsic system, and these can be detected by abnormalities in the activated partial thromboplastin time (APTT). By carrying out both the APTT and the prothrombin time, it is therefore possible to determine whether the defect lies in the initial stages of the intrinsic system or in the components comprising the extrinsic system. If both tests are abnormal, then the defect is in the final common path or there are multiple abnormalities.

Tests for the intrinsic system

Whole-blood clotting time

A simple but insensitive test for the integrity of the intrinsic system is the whole-blood clotting time. Venous blood is taken and quickly placed in a glass tube at 37°C and observed at intervals until clotting occurs. Unfortunately, there is a wide range in the time taken for normal blood to clot by this method; it normally lies between 5 and 11 minutes and in practice the whole-blood clotting time is found to detect only the grosser clotting defects with any degree of certainty. For instance, it will only detect major deficiences of factors VIII and IX. This test is, therefore, rarely performed now.

Activated partial thromboplastin time (APTT)

The wide range of the whole-blood clotting time is due to two variables. First, activation of factor XII by the glass surface is variable and depends on such factors as the type of glass. Secondly, there is a variation in the adsorption and potentiating activities supplied by the platelets, as platelet numbers vary considerably between individuals. The variation due to these two factors can be substantially abolished by the addition of kaolin and phospholipid (partial thromboplastin). Kaolin provides a maximal stimulus for factor XII activation and the phospholipid, a chloroform extract of brain, acts as a platelet substitute. The suggestion that both kaolin and phospholipid should be used in this way was made by Proctor and Rapaport in 1961 and the test is now widely used. The test is simple to carry out. Citrated plasma is obtained and to this is added a mixture of kaolin and phospholipid followed by calcium, and the time taken for the mixture to clot is measured. Prolongation of the clotting time is almost always due to deficiency of factors VIII and IX (provided that deficiency of factor X onwards has been excluded by the prothrombin time) and the test is sufficiently sensitive to detect deficiencies of both these factors when their concentration is reduced to 30% or less of the normal value; that is, it will detect the mild haemophiliacs who only have severe bleeding after minor surgical procedures.

If the APTT is prolonged, it is possible to confirm the diagnosis of either factor VIII or IX deficiency if plasma is available from known cases of haemophilia and factor IX deficiency. Thus if the addition of plasma known to be deficient only in factor VIII does not shorten the clotting time of the sample from the patient under investigation, then the patient must also have a deficiency of factor VIII. Specialized tests are also available for measuring fairly precisely the levels of factor VIII and IX, expressed as a percentage of the normal value; these tests should always be carried out in appropriate cases.

Test for the extrinsic system

The prothrombin time

The test used to measure the integrity of the extrinsic system is the one-stage prothrombin time. This test is carried out by adding factor III (tissue thromboplastin) together with calcium to citrated plasma. The tissues from which factor III is prepared include rabbit, bovine, porcine and human brain; however, human brain thromboplastin is being phased out of use because of the potential hazard that it may contain slow viruses. Reference to Fig. 11.8 shows that factor III feeds into the intrinsic system at the stage $X \rightarrow Xa$ and hence prolongation of the prothrombin time results from deficiencies of I, II, V, VII and X. The prothrombin time is thus a misnomer since deficiency of at least five factors affects the test and prothrombin deficiency alone must be gross before the prothrombin time is prolonged. The test is chiefly sensitive to deficiency of factors V, VII and X. A deficiency of platelets does not affect the prothrombin time.

When measuring the prothrombin time and APTT, it is necessary simultaneously to determine the clotting time using a lyophilized control plasma derived from a pool of hepatitis B-screened and HIV-screened healthy donors. This is because there are always small differences in the activities of the reagents that are used.

When the prothrombin time is used for the control of oral anticoagulant therapy, the results are expressed as the international normalized ratio (INR). This is derived from the prothrombin time ratio (i.e. patient's prothrombin time/mean normal prothrombin time) and a factor determined for each thromboplastin reagent by comparing its activity against an international reference preparation. The value of using the INR is that the same therapeutic ranges apply irrespective of which species the thromboplastin is prepared from.

CONGENITAL COAGULATION DISORDERS

Blood clotting abnormalities can be conveniently divided into two categories, the congenital defects and the acquired defects. This section deals with those that are present from birth.

There is a group of patients who complain of excessive bleeding, either spontaneous or following trauma, usually starting early in life, and who frequently have a family history of a similar condition. These patients usually have one of three diseases, namely, haemophilia, factor IX deficiency or von Willebrand's disease. Out of 187 families with coagulation defects studied by Biggs & MacFarlane (1958), 138 had haemophilia, 20 had factor IX deficiency and 11 had von Willebrand's disease; the patients in the remaining 18 families either had rare deficiencies or had anticoagulants, or were not diagnosed.

Haemophilia (factor VIII deficiency, haemophilia A)

The term haemophilia was first used by Schönlein in 1839 and applies to a life-long tendency to prolonged haemorrhage found only in males and dependent on the transmission of a sex-linked abnormal gene. Apart from the demonstration by Addis in 1911 and Patek & Taylor in 1937 that an active fraction obtained from normal plasma and termed antihaemophilic factor would shorten the clotting time of haemophiliac plasma, there was little understanding of the nature of the defect until the decade of 1950–60.

During this period it was found that there are in fact two diseases within the group of patients who on clinical and genetic grounds had been diagnosed as having haemophilia: patients with factor VIII deficiency and those with factor IX deficiency. The term haemophilia has been retained for factor VIII deficiency, as this is the commoner deficiency, and the terms factor IX deficiency, haemophilia B or Christmas disease (after the name of the first patient) for the other disease.

Deficiency of factor VIII results from an abnormality in the factor VIII gene which lies at the tip of the long arm of the X chromosome. This gene has now been characterized and various abnormalities in the nucleotide sequence have been identified in a number of cases of haemophilia, ranging from single point mutations to large deletions. The disease is thus almost entirely confined to males (XY) since the normal X chromosome in heterozygous females is almost always capable of bringing about adequate factor VIII production; the prevalence of this disorder is about 1 per 10 000 males. Females with haemophilia have been observed extremely rarely and these are either homozygotes for the abnormal gene or are heterozygotes in whom the normal X chromosome has not produced sufficient quantities of factor VIII due to Lyonisation. Daughters of males with haemophilia are obligatory carriers of the gene, since they must inherit the abnormal X chromosome. Sons, on the other hand, are always normal, since they inherit the Y chromosome. A female with a genetic defect on one X chromosome will transmit the disease to half her sons, and half her daughters will become carriers. Patients suspected of having haemophilia should be carefully questioned for a history of a bleeding disorder occurring in the relations on the maternal side as opposed to the paternal side. There is a steady spontaneous mutation rate of the gene responsible for factor VIII production, since approximately one-third of all haemophiliacs have no family history of the disease and this has been corroborated from studies on the genomic DNA.

The factor VIII molecule is a protein with a molecular weight of 80 000 daltons. In the plasma, factor VIII is only found on the von Willebrand factor, which acts as a carrier and prolongs its plasma half-life. Moreover, factor VIII has coagulant activity only when combined with von Willebrand factor. The factor VIII coagulant activity can be measured biologically by its ability to act as a cofactor to factor IX (see Fig. 11.8); the von Willebrand factor can be measured by precipitation with specific antibodies and is, therefore, also known as factor VIII-related antigen.

In haemophilia, it has been found that although factor VIII coagulant activity is greatly depressed, the amount of von Willebrand factor is within normal limits. This observation is important, since it has been possible to make use of this difference for the detection of female carriers of haemophilia. Female carriers on average have half the clotting activity per unit of von Willebrand factor when compared to normals. Discrimination, however, is not perfect and in about 10% of carriers the ratio between the clotting activity and von Willebrand factor content falls within the normal range; thus, those with abnormal ratios can be definitely said to be carriers, but putative carriers with normal ratios cannot be definitely assured that they do not have the abnormal gene.

Prenatal diagnosis of haemophilia can be made by analysis of fetal DNA or blood. DNA can be obtained either by chorionic villus sampling from the ninth week onwards or by amniocentesis between 13 and 16 weeks. The presence or absence of the abnormal gene can be established either directly using appropriate DNA probes or indirectly by restriction-fragment length polymorphism analysis. Fetal blood sampling is done between 18 and 20 weeks. Factor VIII levels are determined in the fetal plasma either on the basis of immunological reactivity or coagulation activity.

Clinical features

The characteristic clinical feature of severe haemophilia is the occurrence of spontaneous bleeding into joints (Fig. 11.10) and less frequently into muscles, these two sites accounting for about 95% of all bleeds requiring treatment (Table 11.1). The presenting symptom is pain in the affected area and this can be very severe. Haemophiliacs rapidly become expert at diagnosing the onset of haemorrhage in its earliest stages, allowing treatment to be initiated at a time when it can be most effective. If not properly treated, bleeding into joints results in crippling deformity. The knees, elbows and ankles are most commonly

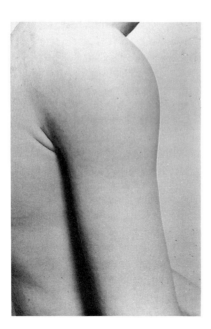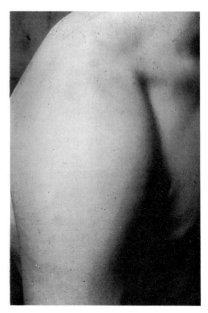

Fig. 11.10   Haemarthrosis of the shoulder joint in a patient with haemophilia A.

affected. Haematuria, epistaxis and gastrointestinal bleeding are less common. Intracranial bleeding is the most common single cause of death, accounting for 25–30% of all deaths; only about one-half of the affected patients have a history of trauma (Eyster *et al* 1978).

The severity of bleeding and mode of presentation is related to the level of plasma factor VIII (Rizza 1977); this relationship is shown in Table 11.2. The severity of the disease often remains constant throughout a family.

Diagnosis

The diagnosis of haemophilia is strongly suggested by the laboratory finding of a normal extrinsic clotting system (normal prothrombin time) and a prolonged activated partial thromboplastin time, since factor VIII deficiency is the commonest abnormality that is found in the initial steps of the intrinsic system. Confirmation can be obtained by showing that the addition of plasma from a

Table 11.1   Frequency of bleeding sites in 207 haemophiliacs. Adapted from Rizza (1977).

Lesion or operation	Percentage
Haemarthroses	79
Muscle haematomas	15
Haematuria	
Epistaxis	
Gastrointestinal bleeding	Each about 1–2%
Dental extraction	Total 6%
Major surgery	

Table 11.2   Relation between plasma factor VIII levels and severity of bleeding. Adapted from Rizza (1977).

Factor VIII level (units/100 ml)	Bleeding symptoms
50	None
25–50	Excessive bleeding after major surgery or serious accident (often not diagnosed until incident occurs)
5–25	Excessive bleeding after minor surgery and injuries
1–5	⎰Severe bleeding after minor surgery ⎱Sometimes spontaneous haemorrhage
0	Spontaneous bleeding into muscles and joints

known case of factor VIII deficiency to the patient's plasma does not correct the clotting defect or can be obtained by a specific assay of factor VIII coagulant activity.

Treatment

Treatment should be given at the earliest sign of spontaneous or post-traumatic bleeding. It should also be given prophylactically if any type of operation is contemplated. Treatment consists of intravenous injections of factor VIII in a concentrated form to maintain plasma factor VIII coagulant activity between 5 and 100% of normal, depending on the severity of the injury or extent of the proposed surgical procedure. In general, the more extensive the bleeding or the degree of trauma, the larger the dose of factor VIII that is required. Two types of concentrated factor VIII preparation are available, cryoprecipitate and freeze-dried factor VIII concentrate. Cryoprecipitate, a relatively impure preparation which is made in a simple manner by the freezing and slow thawing of plasma, is now being replaced by the more expensive but more highly purified freeze-dried material. The large amounts of factor VIII now being used by haemophilia patients has created problems of supply. It has been estimated that approximately 500 000 units of blood are required annually in the UK, which is about 30% of the total number of units available.

Two of the major advantages of the freeze-dried material are that it can be stored at 4°C in a domestic refrigerator and that adequate amounts can be injected in a small volume. This has made it possible for many patients to be treated at home, sometimes by self-administration, thus allowing factor VIII to be injected as soon as symptoms appear. Such early therapy results in both rapid cessation of bleeding and rapid recovery. An excellent account of the value and advantages of home care can be found in the paper of Rizza & Spooner (1977).

Since the half-life of factor VIII in the plasma is about 12 hours, this factor has to be injected twice a day. Frequent assays of factor VIII levels in the plasma may be necessary to ensure that the concentration is being maintained at the appropriate level.

Approximately 5–10% of haemophiliac patients who are repeatedly injected with factor VIII develop antibodies which inhibit its functional activity. These patients require large amounts of factor VIII, or recourse may have to be made to the use of factor VIII of bovine or porcine origin. However the latter can only be used for a short time, since antibodies to these molecules develop rapidly.

Freeze-dried factor VIII preparations are derived from large pools of plasma (500–5000 donations) and several preparations used in the past have contained the human immunodeficiency virus (HIV); as a consequence many haemophiliacs have become infected with HIV. This virus has been virtually eliminated from currently-used preparations by using donors who do not have HIV antibodies and by heat-treating the final product at 80°C for 72 hours, a process known to kill the virus.

The amount of factor VIII required to be given to patients undergoing dental extraction can be reduced by treatment with the antifibrinolytic drug, tranexamic acid. The vasopressin analogue desmopressin (DDAVP) may also be used to increase factor VIII clotting activity in mild or moderate haemophilia.

Factor IX deficiency (haemophilia B, Christmas disease)

The demonstration that there are two genetic defects giving rise to the clinical syndrome of 'haemophilia' was first clearly made by Biggs *et al.* in 1952 and was based on the observation that the addition of plasma from certain 'haemophiliacs' could correct the clotting defect in the plasma of other 'haemophiliacs', which could only be explained by postulating a deficiency of at least two factors. This second factor was soon identified as factor IX. The clinical features and inheritance are identical to factor VIII deficiency, but in general the disease is milder. The incidence varies between different countries; on average, about 20% of those with the clinical syndrome of 'haemophilia' have factor IX deficiency.

The diagnosis can be made by assay of the factor IX level. A freeze-dried factor IX concentrate (actually a prothrombin-complex concentrate containing factors II, VII, IX and X) is available and should be administered intravenously as soon as spontaneous or post-traumatic bleeding starts. Factor IX has a longer half-life in the plasma (24 hours) than factor VIII and hence can be given at less frequent intervals. It has been found that home treatment with factor IX given weekly or fortnightly as a prophylactic measure considerably reduces the incidence of haemorrhage (Rizza & Spooner 1977).

von Willebrand's disease

This rare disease should be mentioned in a discussion on bleeding disorders since its prevalence in Britain is of about the same order as that of factor IX deficiency. It was first described by von Willebrand in 1926 as occurring in several families on islands in the Baltic (Åland Islands). It is characterized by excessive bleeding presenting in infancy which differs from haemophilia in that the defect is not sex-linked. The cause of bleeding is the failure of the platelets to form a haemostatic plug and this failure results either from a reduction in or a complete lack of von Willebrand factor (vWf). This factor is a protein with a molecular weight of 2.7×10^5 daltons and exists in the plasma as a variable-sized polymer ranging from a dimer to a molecule containing 50–100 subunits. It has a dual function: first, it acts as a carrier for factor VIII, one factor VIII molecule being associated with about 1000 vWf subunits; secondly, it is an adhesive molecule which binds platelets to subendothelial tissues. For this purpose there is a binding site on the molecule which binds to collagen and another site which binds to glycoprotein on the platelet membrane. The nature of the genetic defect is now becoming clearer. The gene is present on chromosome 12 and analysis of both the gene and the vWf protein have shown that there is considerable heterogeneity in the structural abnormalities. Most abnormalities result in a simple quantitative reduction in vWf plasma concentration but many different qualitative defects in the molecule also occur.

As vWf acts as a carrier for factor VIII, the reduction in vWf in this disease results in a reduction in factor VIII concentration (usually measured as clotting activity), which may be as low as 5–30% of normal, similar to that found in mild haemophilia. The excessive bleeding in the disease is thus due both to factor VIII deficiency as well as to the failure of the platelets to adhere. An additional finding is that, in contrast to normal platelets, those from people with von Willebrand's disease fail to aggregate in the presence of the antibiotic ristocetin. This observation is the basis of a useful laboratory test for the diagnosis of this disease.

Most patients are heterozygous for the von Willebrand gene and the extent of the bleeding is not great. Spontaneous bleeding is usually confined to mucous membranes and skin and takes the form of epistaxes and ecchymoses. Severe haemorrhage following surgical procedures is not uncommon. Bleeding into joints and muscles is rare except in those patients who are homozygous for the defective gene (Bloom & Peake 1977). Apart from the reduced factor VIII clotting activity, the other abnormalities that are found include a prolonged bleeding time, reduced levels of vWf (factor VIII-related antigen) and impaired ristocetin-induced platelet aggregation; however, there may be periods when the bleeding time is within normal limits. The prolonged bleeding time distinguishes von Willebrand's disease from haemophilia and factor IX deficiency.

Fresh plasma, fresh-frozen plasma or cryoprecipitate are effective in stopping haemorrhage, mainly by correcting the bleeding time but also by increasing factor VIII clotting activity, which continues to increase for many hours after treatment. Factor VIII concentrates are less effective since they have little effect on the bleeding time. For mildly or moderately affected patients, desmopressin (DDAVP) should always be considered before using blood products.

Deficiency of other clotting factors

Single deficiencies of factors other than VIII and IX are very rare, but all possible deficiencies have been found and all except factor XII deficiency give rise to bleeding disorders of varying degrees of severity. The explanation for the absence of excessive haemorrhage in factor XII deficiency is that the activation of the intrinsic pathway can be initiated in the absence of factor XII by the adsorption of factor XI to the surface of activated platelets.

ACQUIRED COAGULATION DISORDERS

The blood clotting factors II, VII, IX and X (collectively known as the prothrombin group or complex) are all produced in the liver and hence a deficiency of these factors occurs in liver disease. Moreover, the final stages in the synthesis of these factors involves a vitamin K-dependent carboxylase, which adds carboxyl (–COOH) groups to the proteins; these groups are necessary for the efficient functioning of the molecules. The coumarin drugs are vitamin K antagonists and their administration results in only partial carboxylation of the prothrombin group of coagulation factors, which are consequently considerably less active than normal in the clotting cascade. Similar abnormalities are seen in vitamin K deficiency, which may be found in patients with intestinal malabsorption and, since bile salts are required for vitamin K absorption, also in patients with biliary obstruction or biliary fistulae. Examination of Fig. 11.8 shows that, except for factor IX, the clotting factors involved are in the extrinsic system and hence the test that is used for detecting these acquired deficiencies is the prothrombin time.

Disseminated intravascular coagulation

Disseminated intravascular coagulation (DIC) describes a process in which there is a generalized activation of the clotting system followed by marked activation of the fibrinolytic system. Acute DIC may be associated with premature separation of the placenta, amniotic fluid embolism or shock and may also be seen in certain bacterial infections such as meningococcaemia, where the endotoxin causes damage to monocytes and vascular endothelium. It is a common complication following intravascular haemolysis of red cells after a mismatched transfusion. The syndrome also occurs occasionally after extensive accidental or surgical trauma, particularly following thoracic operations. Chronic DIC is seen when there is retention of a dead fetus as well as in patients with disseminated carcinoma, lymphoma, leukaemia (especially promyelocytic leukaemia), giant haemangiomas and extensive aortic aneurysms. Other clinical associations are discussed by Deykin (1970).

In those diseases that are associated with DIC, the clotting cascade may be activated in one or both of two ways, namely, by the adsorption and activation of factors XII and XI by damaged vascular endothelium and by the release of tissue factor (factor III) from damaged tissues, monocytes or red cells. Dissemination of factors XIIa, XIa and III in the plasma leads to generalized fibrin deposition on vascular endothelium. If this is sufficiently extensive, there is a reduction of plasma fibrinogen concentration and other clotting factors, which impairs haemostatic activity. As a result of the fibrin formation, the fibrinolytic mechanism is activated by the absorption of plasminogen or tissue plasminogen activator or both to the fibrin. The plasmin then breaks down the fibrin into small fibrin-degradation products (FDP). When fibrin deposition is considerable, the activity of the plasmin results in high concentrations of FDP. This leads to further haemostatic impairment, since FDP inhibit fibrin clot formation by interfering with the polymerization of fibrin monomer. The FDP also interfere with the aggregation of platelets, thus inhibiting their important physiological activity of plugging small vessels. The end result is generalized haemorrhage due to failure of the haemostatic mechanisms (Sharp 1977).

As explained above, the usual clinical manifestation of the generalized activation of the clotting and fibrinolytic systems is haemorrhage. However, occasionally, activation of the clotting mechanism dominates over activation of fibrinolysis and the clinical picture is then that of widespread thrombosis and infarction; thrombi are most frequently found in the microvasculature. The haemorrhagic manifestations may be mild or moderate in chronic DIC but may be so severe in acute DIC as to lead to death. They include petechiae, ecchymoses and bleeding from the nose, mouth, urinary and gastrointestinal tracts and vagina. Haemorrhage may also occur into the pituitary gland, liver, adrenals and brain. Mild hypotension is commonly present in acute DIC and may progress to become more severe and irreversible if not treated in time. Some patients with chronic DIC are asymptomatic because the activation of the clotting and fibrinolytic systems is finely balanced and the production of clotting factors and platelets is sufficiently increased to compensate for their increased consumption.

Diagnosis

This is partly dependent on being aware of the conditions with which DIC is associated. When the syndrome of acute DIC is suspected, the diagnosis is a matter of urgency and it is therefore the tests that can be carried out in the shortest time that are most useful. There are several investigations of value in the diagnosis of acute or chronic DIC.

1   *The platelet count.* Platelets become enmeshed in the fibrin clots on the vascular endothelium and thrombocytopenia is an early and very common sign.

2   *The activated partial thromboplastin time and the prothrombin time.* These are significantly prolonged, due to the depletion of clotting factors.

3   *The fibrinogen concentration.* This can be estimated either on the basis of the time taken for a diluted sample of plasma to clot in the presence of high concentrations of thrombin (Clauss method) or by immunological methods. In the Clauss method, the clotting times are converted to fibrinogen concentrations using a standard curve constructed from the thrombin clotting times given by various dilutions of a standard plasma of known fibrinogen concentration.

4   *The thrombin time.* When the fibrinogen concentration is normal, estimation of the thrombin time is a useful indication of the presence of excessive amounts of FDP. The thrombin time is determined by adding low concentrations of thrombin to citrated plasma and measuring the time for the appearance of a clot. In the presence of FDP, the thrombin time is prolonged due to inhibition of fibrin polymerization.

5   *Estimation of FDP.* The presence of FDP can also be detected by a rapid immunological test using antibody directed against fibrinogen. If latex particles are coated with fibrinogen, they can be agglutinated by anti-fibrinogen and the addition of serum containing FDP will inhibit this agglutination; the greater the FDP level, the greater the inhibition.

Treatment

Since the activation of the clotting system is the primary initiating stimulus and fibrinolysis is mainly a secondary phenomenon, treatment is aimed at preventing further coagulation by removal of the initiating cause (e.g. when it occurs in obstetric practice, rapid and non-traumatic vaginal delivery stops the clotting process). Whilst the initiating cause is being dealt with, patients with acute DIC should be supported with transfusions of blood, fresh-frozen plasma and platelet concentrates in order to restore blood volume and to replace clotting factors and platelets.

INVESTIGATION OF A PATIENT WITH ABNORMAL BLEEDING

The investigation of most patients with a congenital or acquired haemostatic defect can be undertaken in any well-equipped haematology laboratory. However, the diagnosis of the rarer congenital coagulation abnormalities requires specialized laboratories. This is because many of the requisite tests are complex and difficult to carry out reliably and accurately unless performed reasonably frequently.

A most important step in the diagnostic process is the taking of a good history from the patient (Biggs 1968). The physician should ask, amongst others, the following questions: Has the patient ever bled excessively in the past and have any relatives bled excessively? More specifically, has the patient had tonsillectomy, major abdominal or orthopaedic surgery or dental extractions in the past and if so was there any abnormal bleeding? The excellent paper of Ingram (1977) should be consulted for a more detailed discussion of the taking of the patient's own, and family, history. The relationship between the type of bleeding and the nature of the haemostatic defect has been discussed earlier (p. 160).

The screening tests that are useful in investigating a patient who gives a history of excessive bleeding are the following:

Examination of a blood film
Platelet count
Bleeding time
Prothrombin time
Activated partial thromboplastin time
Thrombin time
Fibrinogen assay

If any of these tests is found to be abnormal, further specialized tests may be necessary.

OBJECTIVES IN LEARNING

1 To know the morphology and function of platelets and the relationship between the number of platelets in the peripheral blood and the extent of abnormal bleeding.

2 To know about (a) the diseases associated with a failure of platelet production; and (b) the diseases associated with a shortened platelet life span, especially idiopathic thrombocytopenia purpura.

3 To know the main sequence of events in both the intrinsic and extrinsic clotting pathways.

4 To know the principles underlying the tests for the intrinsic system (whole blood clotting time and activated partial thromboplastin time) and for the extrinsic system (prothrombin time).

5   To know the mode of inheritance, clinical presentation, method of diagnosis and treatment of haemophilia, factor IX deficiency and von Willebrand's disease.

6   To know the effects of coumarin drugs, vitamin-K deficiency and liver disease on the clotting mechanisms and the method of diagnosis of such acquired abnormalities of coagulation.

7   To know the alterations in the haemostatic and fibrinolytic mechanisms associated with disseminated intravascular coagulation.

8   To know the principles of investigation of a patient suspected of having a haemostatic defect.

REFERENCES

Ackroyd J.F. (1962) The immunological basis of purpura due to drug hypersensitivity. *Proc Roy Soc Med* **55**: 437

Addis T. (1911) The pathogenesis of hereditary haemophilia. *J. Pathol. Bacteriol.* **15**, 427

Aster R.H. (1972) Platelet sequestration studies in man. *Br. J. Haematol.* **22**, 259

Barkhan P. (1966) Platelet survival studies in man with diisopropylphosphorofluoridate (DF^{32}P)*Br. J. Haematol.* **12: 25.**

Beresford C.H. (1988) Antithrombin III deficiency. *Blood Reviews* **2**: 239

Biggs R. (1968) The detection of defects in blood coagulation. *Br. J. Haematol.* **15**: 115

Biggs R., Douglas A.S., MacFarlane R.G., Dacie J.V., Pitney W.R., Merskey C., O'Brien J.R. (1952) Christmas disease: a condition previously mistaken for haemophilia. *Br. Med. J.* **2**: 1378

Biggs R., MacFarlane R.G. (1958) Haemophilia and related conditions: a survey of 187 cases. *Br. J. Haematol.* **4**: 1

Bloom A.L., Peake I.R. (1977) Factor VIII and its inherited disorders. *Br. Med. Bull.* **33**: 219

Deykin D. (1970) The clinical challenge of disseminated intravascular coagulation. *New Engl. J. Med.* **283**: 636

Doan C.A., Bouroncle B.A., Wiseman B.K. (1960) Idiopathic and secondary thrombocytopenic purpura: clinical study and evaluation of 381 cases over a period of 28 years. *Ann. Int. Med.* **53**: 861

Editorial (1971) Platelet transfusions. *Br. Med. J.* **i**: 2

Eyster M.E., Gill F.M., Blatt P.M., Hilgartner M.W., Ballard J.O., Kinney T.R. *et al.*(1978) Central nervous system bleeding in haemophiliacs. *Blood* **51**: 1179

Gaydos L. A., Freireich E. J., Mantel N. (1962) The quantitative relation between platelet count and haemorrhage in patients with acute leukaemia. *New Engl. J. Med* **266**: 905

Harker L.A., Slichter S. J. (1972) The bleeding time as a screening test for evaluation of platelet function. *New Engl. J. Med.* **287**: 155

Harrington W.J., Minnich V., Hollingsworth J.W., Moore C.V. (1951) Demonstration of a thrombocytopenic factor in the blood of patients with thrombocytopenia purpura. *J. Lab. Clin. Med.* **38**: 1

Ingram G.I.C. (1977) Investigation of a long-standing bleeding tendency. *Br. Med. Bull.* **33**: 261

Lusher J.M., Zeulzer W.W. (1966) Idiopathic thrombocytopenic purpura in childhood. *J. Pediatrics* **68**: 971

MacFarlane R.G. (1964) An enzyme cascade in the blood-clotting mechanism, and its function as a biochemical amplifier. *Nature* **202**: 498

MacFarlane R.G. (1967) Russell's viper venom. *Br. J. Haematol.* **13**: 437

MacFarlane R.G. (1969) The development of a theory of blood coagulation. *Proc. R. Soc. B.* **173**: 261

Manucci P.M., Tripodi A. (1988) Inherited factors in thrombosis. *Blood Reviews* **2**: 27

Mustard J.F., Packham M.A. (1977) Normal and abnormal haemostasis. *Br. Med. Bull.* **33**: 187

Najean Y., Ardaillon N. (1971) The sequestration site of platelets in idiopathic thrombocytopenia purpura: its correlation with the results of splenectomy. *Br. J. Haematol.* **21**: 153

Patek A.J., Taylor F.A.L. (1937) Hemophilia: some properties of substance obtained from normal human plasma effective in accelerating coagulation of hemophilic blood. *J. Clin. Invest.* **16**: 113

Proctor R., Rapaport S.I. (1961) The partial thromboplastin time with kaolin. *Am. J. Clin. Pathol.* **36**: 212

Rizza C.R. (1977) Clinical management of haemophilia. *Br. Med. Bull.* **33**: 225

Rizza C.R., Spooner R.J.D. (1977) Home treatment of haemophilia and Christmas disease: five years experience. *Br. J. Haematol.* **37**: 53

Schulman I (1964) Management of idiopathic thrombocytopenic purpura. *Pediatrics* **33**: 979

Serpick A.A. (1965) Platelet transfusion therapy. *J. Am. Med. Ass.* **192**: 625

Sharp A.A. (1977) Diagnosis and management of disseminated intravascular coagulation. *Br. Med. Bull.* **33**: 265

RECOMMENDED READING

Esnouf M.P. (1977) Biochemistry of blood coagulation. *Br. Med. Bull.* **33**: 213

Mackie M.J., Douglas A.S. (1976) Anticoagulants. *Br. J. Hosp. Med.* **16**: 118

Marcus A.J. (1969) Platelet functions I, II and III. *New Engl. J. Med.* **280**: 1213, 1278 and 1330 (review articles)

Packham M.A., Mustard J.F. (1977) Clinical pharmacology of platelets. *Blood* **50**: 555

Chapter 12
Blood Transfusion

One of the main problems in the transfusion of blood is the avoidance of immunological reactions resulting from the differences in the chemical constituents of the red cells between donor and recipient. Blood groups have arisen because mutations have occurred in the genes controlling the surface constituents of the red cells. These alterations in the surface structures have not affected the function of the red cell but when the red cells of a donor are transfused into a recipient who lacks these surface structures, the recipient treats them as foreign substances and produces antibodies against them. There are at least a dozen major sites on the chromosomes where there are genes responsible for red-cell surface constituents and each of these sites is responsible for a different blood-group system. Although all the systems have given rise to transfusion difficulties (and in fact this is how many have been recognized), fortunately only two, the ABO and Rh systems, are of major importance.

ABO SYSTEM

The ABO system has three allelomorphic genes, *A*, *B* and *O*. The first two genes are responsible for converting a basic substance, H, present in every red cell, into A or B substances, thus converting the cells into groups A or B. The *O* gene has no known effect on the H substance, so that group O red cells simply contain H substance. H substance is a carbohydrate chain attached to lipid or protein in the red-cell membrane. A terminal sugar molecule is attached to this chain which determines the antigenic specificity, *N*-acetylgalactosamine in the case of A antigen and galactose in the case of B antigen. The *A* and *B* genes each code for the two different enzymes (glycosyltransferases) which attach these terminal groups. The *O* gene has no recognized product. The three allelomorphic genes combine in pairs to give six possible genotypes, *AA*, *AO*, *BB*, *BO*, *AB* and *OO*. In determining the blood group of a person, it is necessary to distinguish between genotype and phenotype. Genotype refers to the specific genes that the person carries, whereas the phenotype refers to the observed characteristics, that is, the agglutination reactions brought about by the appropriate antibodies. Determination of the ABO blood group of a person is carried out using only two antibodies, anti-A and anti-B, but not with anti-O, since O substance does not exist. Genotypes can only be determined by family studies; e.g. the genotype *AO* and *AA* cannot be distinguished by agglutinating antibodies and both of these genotypes will be classified as the phenotype A. Thus, only four phenotypes are distinguished, namely A, B, AB and O. As the phenotype A includes the genotypes *AA* and *AO*, it follows that a mating between two people of phenotype A can produce a child of group O, if both parents are genotypically *AO*. The same principle holds for the phenotype B. (Note that it is a convention to print the genotype in italics and the phenotype in Roman letters.)

The frequency of the ABO groups differs in different populations and in Britain it is approximately: group O: 46%, A: 42%, B: 9% and AB: 3%.

There are several subgroups (such as A_1, A_2, etc) within both the A and B groups, resulting from minor biochemical differences in the basic A and B substances. These are of considerable interest to the geneticist but are of no clinical significance. The antibodies anti-A_1 and anti-H are only very rarely found in patients requiring transfusion, and even when they are found, are usually too weak to lead to *in vivo* destruction of red cells containing A_1 or H substance.

Substances with antigenic properties closely similar to those of A and B are widely distributed in nature and are found in many animals and bacteria. Absorption of these substances from the gut is presumed to give rise to the production of anti-A and anti-B in the plasma of those who do not possess the substances on their red cells. Because of the presence of these antibodies it is necessary to transfuse blood with the same ABO group as that of the recipient. As group O cells do not react either with anti-A or anti-B, people of group O came to be known as 'universal donors'. However, this is a dangerous concept, because group O people have anti-A and anti-B in their plasma, and in a small number of people these antibodies may be very potent so that a transfusion of 500 ml of group O blood may contain sufficient anti-A or anti-B to react with the recipient's cells and bring about their destruction.

RH SYSTEM

The Rh system derives its name from the findings of Landsteiner and Wiener (1940) that the antibody produced in rabbits by the injection of red cells from the Rhesus monkey would agglutinate the red cells of 85% of humans (Rh-positive) but not of the remaining 15% (Rh-negative). It was quickly discovered that a similar antibody could also be found in the plasma of humans after blood transfusion and in the plasma of mothers who had given birth to a child with haemolytic disease of the newborn. Several other antibodies were found in humans which were clearly recognizing antigens within the Rh system and in 1943 Fisher put forward the well-known theory that there are three allelomorphic pairs of genes within the Rh system, C and c, D and d, E and e, each gene being responsible for producing a different protein molecule on the surface of the red cell, termed C and c, D, E and e. These molecules are antigenic when blood is transfused into a recipient lacking the molecule on their red cells. The d molecule does not exist and the gene may be defective in some way.

People who were originally labelled as Rh-positive on the old nomenclature have the D antigen on their red cells. Thus, people who are either homozygous *DD*, or heterozygous *Dd*, are Rh-positive while those who are *dd* are Rh-negative. The three genes are on chromosome 1 (either C or c, D or d, E or e) and lie very close together since no crossing-over has ever been found. They are thus always inherited as a specific combination, the three most common being *CDe*, *cde* and *cDE*. As one of the chromosomes in each chromosome pair is derived from the father and one from the mother, the final genotype might be *CDe/cde* which is the commonest combination. Rh-negative blood-transfusion donors are always *cde/cde*.

Differentiation of people into the Rh-positive and Rh-negative groups is carried out only with anti-D, since anti-d does not exist. Use of an antibody of only one specificity means that homozygous *DD* people cannot be differentiated from heterozygous *Dd* people. However, since all the genes of the Rh system are inherited in specific combinations, determination of the presence or absence of the other antigens, (C, c, E and e), especially when combined with family studies, can almost always differentiate *DD* from *Dd*. This assessment is sometimes required to determine whether an Rh-negative mother who has anti-D in her plasma can conceive an Rh-negative child by an Rh-positive father; this can only happen if the father is *Dd*.

Clinically, only the D antigen and anti-D are important. The reason for this is that the D antigen is a much more potent antigen than the others (C, c, E or e) in the sense that it stimulates antibody production with far greater frequency than any of the other antigens in the Rh system. Thus, an Rh-negative person (i.e. *cde/cde*) has over a 50% chance of developing anti-D after the transfusion of one unit of Rh-positive blood, whereas the 'c' antigen will only provoke anti-c production in 2% of people lacking this antigen (Mollison *et al.*1987). It is thus important that Rh-negative people receive Rh-negative blood. On the other hand, the risk from giving Rh-negative blood (*cde/cde*) to an Rh-positive person without the 'c' antigen (for instance whose genotype is *CDe/CDe*) is very small. Nevertheless, it should not be forgotten that the 'c' antigen on Rh-negative red cells is capable of stimulating anti-c production in a few people and that this anti-c will not only demand careful cross-matching at a subsequent transfusion, but can cross the placenta and produce haemolytic disease of the newborn in an infant with the 'c' antigen on its cells.

OTHER BLOOD-GROUP SYSTEMS

Other blood-group antibodies, which are sometimes a problem during blood transfusion, include the following: anti-K (Kell system), anti-Fy^a (Duffy system) and anti-Jk^a(Kidd system). The systems are named after the people in whom the antibody was first detected. Unless an antibody against one of the antigens in these systems is present in the recipient, there is no need to take these groups into account in selecting donor blood. The chief reason for this is that the antigens of these systems are 'poor' antigens and infrequently stimulate antibody production. Thus, compared to the D antigen, their relative potency in stimulating antibody production is 10–1000 times less.

COMPATIBILITY

The purpose of cross-matching blood before transfusion is to ensure there is no antibody present in the recipient's plasma which will react with any antigen on the donor's cells. The basic technique for detecting the antibody, i.e. agglutination of the red cells by antibody, has remained unchanged for over one hundred years. Agglutination was first observed in 1869 by Creite in Goettingen when he found that serum of one animal would agglutinate red cells of another species; the fact that the agglutinating agents were antibodies was not discovered until 1890. The process of agglutination can be divided into two stages:

1 the reaction between antibody and the antigen on the red-cell surface;

2 the clumping together of these red cells as a result of the presence of antibody on their surface.

Unfortunately, many red-cell antibodies are unable to bring about the second stage of agglutination without additional 'help' and thus from a practical point of view antibodies can be divided into agglutinating and non-agglutinating types. The ability of antibodies to agglutinate depends partly on the molecular structure of the antibody. Most IgM antibodies (i.e. those with a molecular weight of 900 000 daltons) can bring about agglutination. By contrast, only some IgG antibodies (molecular weight 160 000 daltons), notably anti-A and B, can bring about agglutination; most IgG antibodies in the other blood group systems do not do so. The Rh blood-group system would probably have been discovered long before 1940 if the IgG anti-D had been an agglutinating antibody. The non-agglutinating antibodies are sometimes referred to as 'incomplete'.

Two methods are available for converting non-agglutinating into agglutinating antibodies: the addition of albumin and the use of enzymes. The addition of 20% albumin to the mixture of red cells and antibody or the treatment of red cells with proteolytic enzymes such as papain, prior to reaction with antibody, will allow agglutination to take place in most instances. However, the most satisfactory test for the presence of non-agglutinating antibodies in a cross-match is the antiglobulin test.

The antiglobulin test

The antiglobulin test was first discovered by Moreschi in 1908 but was forgotten and rediscovered by Coombs, Mourant and Race in 1945. At the time that the test was devised, antibodies were thought to be γ-globulins and the five classes of immunoglobulins, IgG, IgM, IgA, IgD and IgE, had not been identified. Under the new nomenclature, the basic constituent of an antiglobulin serum is anti-IgG and is obtained by injecting human IgG into animals. Antiglobulin serum is able to bring about agglutination by combining with IgG antibodies on the red-cell surface. As anti-IgG antibodies are bivalent, they can combine with one IgG molecule on one red cell and with another IgG molecule on another cell and hence hold the red cells together as agglutinates.

The antiglobulin test can be used in two ways. It can be used to detect antibody already on the patient's cells *in vivo* as in some types of immune haemolytic anaemia and haemolytic disease of the newborn. Red cells from the patient or from cord blood are washed to remove free IgG, which would otherwise react with and neutralise the antiglobulin. After washing, antiglobulin serum is added and agglutination takes place (the direct antiglobulin test). Alternatively, the test can be used to detect the presence of non-agglutinating antibody in plasma or serum, as in the cross-matching of blood for transfusion. In this case, serum from the patient requiring transfusion is incubated with red cells from the donor blood. Any antibody present in the recipient's serum which is active against the donor's cells will combine with the latter and after washing the cells, addition of antiglobulin serum will bring about agglutination (the indirect antiglobulin test).

Procedure for obtaining compatible blood

The ABO and Rh group of the recipient must first be determined. The ABO group is determined by the addition of agglutinating anti-A and anti-B to the red cells. Since it is important to transfuse blood of the correct ABO group, the grouping is checked by determining whether anti-A or anti-B is present in the recipient's serum by adding the serum to known group A and B cells; group A blood always contains anti-B in the plasma, group B blood has anti-A and group O has anti-A and anti-B. The Rh group is determined using an agglutinating IgM anti-D or by using IgG anti-D combined with the antiglobulin test.

Donor blood of the appropriate ABO and Rh group is then selected. The usual practice is for the organizations collecting the blood (i.e. the Regional Blood Transfusion Centres) to determine the ABO and Rh group of the donor blood. Before this blood can be transfused, cross-matching must be carried out. The purpose of the cross-match is partly to ensure that there have been no errors in the determination of the ABO group of the donor and recipient, and partly to ensure that no antibodies are present in the recipient which react with the donor's red cells. Since the antibodies in the recipient's plasma may be agglutinating or non-agglutinating, two tests are carried out. First, a test for agglutinating antibodies in which the patient's own serum is added to the donor's cells and incubated at 37°C. The cells are then examined for agglutination. Secondly, a test for non-agglutinating antibodies, i.e. the antiglobulin test, using the patient's serum and the donor's cells.

In most transfusion laboratories, it is now usual for the sera of all recipients to be screened for the presence of antibodies such as anti-K, anti-Fy[a] and anti-Jk[a], using a panel of red cells of known phenotype, whenever time permits. If screening is not carried out, these antibodies will be discovered in the final stages of a cross-matching procedure, using the antiglobulin test. When an antibody turns up during the serum screen, its specificity has first to be identified and then donor blood lacking the appropriate antigen must be found. As this takes time, cross-matching should always be carried out at least 1 day in advance of planned surgery in order to allow for this possibility.

Rh-negative donor blood is not always available for Rh-negative recipients and the question arises whether it is safe to give Rh-positive blood. Rh-negative males, especially elderly males, may receive Rh-positive blood provided care is taken to search for anti-D if subsequent transfusions are given. In women past the menopause the procedure is less safe because there is always the possibility, admittedly small, that they may have received a primary stimulus with D antigen from an Rh-positive fetus and the anti-D in the plasma may be below a detectable level. Transfusion of Rh-positive blood would then provoke a secondary response of anti-D production leading to a delayed transfusion reaction after a few days. Rh-positive blood must never be given to Rh-negative females of child-bearing age for fear of stimulating anti-D production and thus of producing haemolytic disease of the newborn in a subsequent pregnancy.

Ensuring that the patient receives the correct blood

Experience has shown that the most frequent cause of giving incompatible blood is incorrect labelling of samples, confusion between recipients with the same name, or failure to check from the label on the blood bag that the blood being transfused is the blood that has been cross-matched with the patient. Incompatible transfusions are only rarely due to mismatching of blood in the laboratory. Responsibility for giving the wrong blood usually lies with the person who takes the sample of the recipient's blood for cross-matching or with the person who sets up the transfusion. When taking blood for cross-matching, great care should be taken that this is correctly labelled. The blood should be put into a container which is already labelled with the patient's name and hospital number and the label should be signed by the person who takes the sample. Requests for blood, however urgent, must be made in writing on the appropriate request form. When the donor blood has been found to be compatible, the laboratory staff place a compatibility label on it, stating the patient's name, hospital number and the serial number of that particular bag of blood. The person who sets up the transfusion is then finally responsible for ensuring that the patient's name and hospital number on the compatibility label apply to the patient who is being transfused and also that the serial number on the compatibility label is the same as the serial number of the bag of blood.

It cannot be too frequently emphasized that the commonest cause of incompatible transfusions is the carelessness of those responsible for setting up the transfusions. The patient must be particularly closely observed during the first 20 minutes following the start of the transfusion, to detect any evidence of a reaction due to incompatible or infected blood. This precaution is extremely important, since symptoms of an incompatible transfusion usually appear within this time and, if the transfusion is stopped at an early stage, the chance of a fatal outcome is reduced.

DONOR BLOOD

Donor blood (approximately 420 ml) is mixed with 120 ml of citrate–phosphate–dextrose with adenine (CPD-adenine), a solution found empirically to give good preservation of the blood. If the blood is stored at 4 °C, 80% of the cells are still viable after 28 days, the remaining 20% being removed from the circulation by the reticuloendothelial system within a few hours of transfusion. After 35 days of storage the percentage of viable cells falls off fairly rapidly, so that the blood is not used after this period of time. When plasma is removed from CPD-adenine blood for the purpose of preparing fresh-frozen plasma or plasma products, the red cells may be transfused after storage for up to 35 days, if stored in a solution containing saline, adenine, glucose and mannitol (SAG-M).

TRANSFUSION IN ACUTE HAEMORRHAGE AND CHRONIC ANAEMIAS

Patients with acute haemorrhage (i.e. loss of red cells and plasma) should be transfused with whole blood or with red cells suspended in SAG-M. If more than four units of red cells in SAG-M have to be transfused, Purified Protein Fraction (90–98% albumin) must also be given. Plasma-reduced blood with a PCV of about 65% or concentrated red cells in SAG-M should be used when patients with a severe chronic anaemia have to be transfused, as such patients have an increased plasma volume and are prone to develop circulatory overload. Further steps which should be taken to minimize this complication are to administer a diuretic before the transfusion and to ensure that the rate of transfusion is slow.

HAZARDS OF BLOOD TRANSFUSION

Blood transfusion has become such a commonplace procedure that the hazards of transfusion are frequently overlooked. The actual mortality resulting directly from transfusion is difficult to estimate and undoubtedly varies from region to region. The main causes of death nowadays are post-transfusion hepatitis and incompatible transfusion; bacterial infection, circulatory overload and other causes are only to blame in a minority of cases.

The unfavourable reactions to transfusion are either immediate, in which case they are due to pyrogens, allergens, bacteria, circulatory overloading or incompatible blood, or the reactions are delayed; in which case they are due to the transmission of diseases such as hepatitis, malaria or syphilis.

The recognition of these hazards has been a lengthy process. Before the discovery of the ABO blood-groups, haemolytic reactions due to this blood-group system were frequent and hence transfusions were few. When ABO incompatibility was eliminated, one of the first hazards to be recognized was the transfer of syphilis. With the increasing use of blood after the introduction of citrate as an anticoagulant in 1914, reactions due to allergens and pyrogens became recognized. It was in 1943 that the first reports of transmission of hepatitis were made (Ministry of Health Memorandum 1943) and it was during this and the following decade that reactions due to blood groups other than the ABO group were described. The most recent addition to the hazards of transfusion is the transmission of the human immunodeficiency virus (HIV).

Haemolytic reactions due to incompatible red cells

With advances in blood-grouping and crossing-matching techniques, haemolytic reactions have now become rare; Ramgren et al. (1958) assessed the incidence in Sweden to be about 1 in 5000 during the 5 years of 1951–1955. Mollison (1979), surveying more recent figures, came to a similar conclusion. The number of mismatched transfusions, however, is certainly greater than this, since the distribution of the ABO groups is such that, if either donor or recipient is mis-identified and the wrong blood given, there is only a 1 in 3 chance of that blood being incompatible (e.g. group A recipient misidentified as group O and receiving group O blood would not have a haemolytic reaction, whereas the reverse would lead to incompatibility). This means that the incidence of mismatched (but not necessarily incompatible) transfusions may be as high as 1 in 1500.

The symptoms that are found after a transfusion of incompatible blood depend on whether the transfused cells suffer intravascular lysis or whether they are phagocytosed by the reticuloendothelial system and subjected to extravascular lysis. Intravascular lysis leads to haemoglobinaemia and haemoglobinuria and is almost always due to the action of anti-A or anti-B which bring about lysis in conjunction with the complement system. Usually within a few minutes of transfusing ABO incompatible blood, there is a feeling of heat along the vein used for transfusion, flushing of the face, pain in the lumbar region and chest, and chilliness. This is followed by fever. These effects are thought to be due to the release of the complement fragments C3a and C5a, since the complement sequence is known to be activated following the combination of anti-A with A red cells. If the reaction is severe, there is circulatory collapse and sometimes extensive haemorrhage due to the release of clotting factor III and plasminogen activator from red cells, which results in disseminated intravascular coagulation and fibrinolysis. If the patient survives the initial reaction, there is about a 10% chance of developing oliguria or anuria. The mechanism by which this is brought about is still disputed, but it is probable that an important factor is the toxic action of high concentrations of haemoglobin on the renal tubules. The immediate treatment of a mismatched transfusion would therefore be to promote diuresis with frusemide. When deaths do occur, they are usually the result either of severe disseminated intravascular coagulation or of renal failure. If the latter is correctly treated with due attention to water, electrolyte and protein intake, the mortality from renal damage should be low. The overall mortality following ABO incompatibility is probably of the order of 10%. Wallace (1977) reported four deaths from 40 incompatible transfusions in a survey involving 130 000 recipients of blood.

When blood transfusion is followed by extravascular destruction of red cells there are usually only chills and fever occurring one or more hours after the start of the transfusion. The most common antibody causing extravascular destruction is anti-D. This type of incompatibility is almost never followed by renal failure.

Another type of incompatibility is the delayed haemolytic transfusion reaction. This occurs when a recipient has been previously immunized by transfusion or pregnancy but in whom the antibody in the plasma has become too weak to be identified. Following the transfusion, a secondary immunological response takes place and the antibody titre rapidly rises, bringing about haemolysis, usually about seven days later. Typically, the patient develops anaemia, fever, jaundice and sometimes haemoglobinuria. The incidence of this type of reaction may be as high as 1 in 4000 recipients (Pineda et al. 1978).

Pyrexia due to pyrogens, leucocyte antibodies and platelet antibodies

Pyrogens were once a common cause of reactions. They are soluble polysaccharides produced by bacteria and are present in preparations of distilled water, citrate, dextrose and sodium chloride. Contamination by pyrogens has been reduced by strict control during manufacture of the anticoagulants. Chills and fever start 30–60 minutes after the onset of the transfusion and can be mitigated or abolished by aspirin. Febrile reactions may also be caused by the presence of anti-HLA, granulocyte-specific and platelet-specific antibodies in the recipient as the result of sensitization during pregnancy or repeated transfusion. Since pyrogen reactions are now a rarity, febrile reactions should always suggest the possibility that incompatible red cells, leucocytes or platelets have been transfused.

Immediate-type hypersensitivity

Hypersensitivity reactions may occur soon after the transfusion of blood or plasma. The antibodies involved are often unknown but some severe reactions are caused by antibodies against IgA present in recipients lacking IgA who have previously become sensitized to this Ig. In mild cases, the only manifestation may be urticarial wheals, erythema, maculo-papular rash or periorbital oedema. In the more severe reactions, hypotension may occur; bronchial spasm and laryngeal oedema are rare. Mild reactions probably occur in about 1–3% of transfusions and can be treated with antihistamines. Severe reactions are very infrequent (1:20 000) and these require the administration of hydrocortisone and adrenalin.

The cause of these reactions is uncertain, but thought to be the release of the complement components, C3a and C5a, and also the release of leukotrienes.

Bacterial contamination

Transfusion of infected blood is fortunately rare, but when it does occur is frequently lethal. The low incidence is due entirely to the most painstaking precautions to keep solutions, storage containers and transfusion equipment sterile. However, there is one source of infection that is difficult to eliminate and that is the introduction of organisms from the skin during blood donation, despite careful attempts to disinfect the skin. Skin contaminants entering donor blood are usually staphylococci which fortunately do not grow at 4°C; as many as 2% of all donor blood may be found to have these organisms within the first 24 hours, but they are killed off during storage and are only rarely found after 3 weeks' storage.

Occasionally, however, Gram-negative bacteria enter donor blood and these will grow slowly at 4°C (doubling time about 8 hours), although they grow preferentially at 20°C. In 2–3 weeks at 4°C, growth can be sufficient to cause a lethal reaction and it is usually this type of organism that is found in the fatal cases. The growth rate of these bacteria is considerably speeded up if the blood is brought to and kept at room temperature. The risks of transfusing infected blood can thus be minimised by keeping blood at 4°C until the moment of transfusion. One or more deaths from infected blood are usually reported each year in the UK. The chief signs of transfusion of infected blood are the rapid onset of pyrexia and circulatory collapse. Haemorrhage due to disseminated intravascular coagulation may occur.

Circulatory overload

Circulatory overload with consequent cardiac failure can easily be brought about by the too rapid transfusion of blood, especially in the elderly and in those who have been severely anaemic for some time. The first signs are dyspnoea, a dry cough, crepitations at the lung bases and a rise in jugular venous pressure. If there is any indication of overload, the transfusion must be stopped and venesection may be necessary. The risk of circulatory overload can be minimized in patients with severe anaemia by giving only 250 ml of concentrated red cells (i.e. a unit of blood with most of the plasma-citrate removed) and restricting the rate of transfusion to 1 ml/kg body weight/hour. If the patient is only mildy anaemic and has normal cardiac function, 1 litre can be safely transfused over a 5 hour period. This is about one drop per second with the standard giving sets.

Citrate toxicity

Citrate toxicity may develop and can cause death if large volumes of stored blood have to be given very rapidly. It is due to the reduction in ionized calcium in the patient's plasma. The signs are gross skeletal muscle tremors and prolongation of the QT interval in the ECG. If more than 2 litres are given every 20 minutes then each litre should be accompanied by 1g of calcium gluconate. The potassium which leaks out of red cells during storage is probably only dangerous when excess citrate is present in the recipient's plasma.

Transmission of disease

Post-transfusion hepatitis

Viral hepatitis is a most important complication of the transfusion of blood because of the relatively high incidence of virus carriers in certain populations, the tendency for a chronic liver infection to develop in a substantial proportion of patients and, in the case of hepatitis B, a high fatality rate from fulminant hepatic failure.

Several viruses are known to cause hepatitis when infection occurs naturally (i.e. not by the intravenous route); these include hepatitis A and hepatitis B (HB) viruses, cytomegalovirus, herpes simplex virus, Epstein-Barr virus and an obscure virus or group of viruses termed for convenience 'non-A, non-B'. Of these, only the hepatitis B and the non-A, non-B viruses play any significant part in post-transfusion hepatitis.

Hepatitis B

Knowledge of the hepatitis B virus has been greatly expanded since the discovery that the abnormal serum protein known as Australia antigen (first found in the serum of an Australian aborigine) is the surface coat of the HB virus. The virus has been identified by electron microscopy as a 42 nm particle (the Dane particle) and its presence in serum can be demonstrated by a sensitive radioimmunoassay test, involving the use of the antibody against the surface antigen, HBsAg. The prevalence of HB virus in symptomless subjects (as recognized by finding the HBsAg) varies between different populations, being as low as 0.1% in volunteer donors in the UK and USA but as high as 15% in certain parts of the world. The usual mode of transmission of the virus in the general population is probably through close contact. It has been suggested that HB may also be transmitted sexually, as high rates of infection are found in homosexual men and prostitutes. The identification and elimination of all donor blood containing detectable HBsAg has brought about a very considerable reduction in the incidence of hepatitis B. The sensitivity of the tests, however, is not sufficient to eliminate all donors who are carriers.

Non-A, non-B hepatitis

Post-transfusion hepatitis (PTH) in which the known hepatitis agents, hepatitis B, cytomegalovirus and EBV have been excluded is known as 'non-A, non-B'. There is evidence that more than one virus may be involved. Substantial progress has been made recently in that viral RNA has been identified which encodes for a protein that reacts with antibody obtained from a high proportion of patients with chronic non-A, non-B hepatitis. This virus has been designated as hepatitis C (Choo *et al.* 1989). About 15% of patients with PTH are negative for hepatitis B and hepatitis C.

Now that hepatitis B virus has been largely eliminated from donor blood, the non-A, non-B viruses are the main agents of PTH. Recent surveys have shown that the incidence of PTH varied widely between different countries, values varying from an incidence of 2% in Australia to 40% in Japan. It is thought that 80% or more of the cases are due to the non-A, non-B viruses. Although no large-scale study has been made in the UK, the incidence of PTH in the 1980s is thought to be about 2–3%.

Although prepared from pools of donated plasma, several of the currently available factor VIII, factor IX and fibrinogen concentrates carry only a minimal risk of transmitting hepatitis B and non-A, non-B virus. This reduction in risk has been achieved not only by the screening of donors for HBsAg and for elevated alanine aminotransferase (a possible surrogate marker for non-A, non-B hepatitis) but also by the use of better fractionation procedures (e.g. the use of monoclonal immunoabsorption) and by heat-treatment of the product to inactivate virus. Fortunately albumin and immunoglobulin preparations are free of hepatitis viruses.

Clinical aspects

It can be seen from Fig. 12.1 that the time of onset of overt hepatitis varies from about 2 weeks to 6 months after the transfusion. For every case of icteric hepatitis, it is generally accepted that there are several times as many cases of anicteric hepatitis. Thus, most of those who develop the disease are only mildly ill or may have no symptoms. The hepatitis can only be recognized in these patients by a rise in the plasma levels of liver enzymes such as aspartate and alanine transaminase. A substantial proportion of older icteric patients with post-transfusion HB die of fulminant hepatitis, perhaps because of the large load

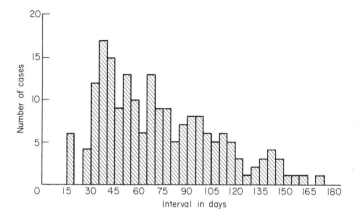

Fig. 12.1   The interval from transfusion to onset of hepatitis in 195 patients receiving blood or blood products on a single day. Adapted from Mosley (1965)

of virus entering the body. The mortality rate almost certainly varies with the strain of the virus and is around 10–20%. For example, Mosley (1965) reported an 11% mortality in patients who developed icteric hepatitis. By contrast, patients with non-A, non-B post-transfusion hepatitis only occasionally suffer from fulminant hepatitis (Seeff *et al.* 1977). Nevertheless, although non-A, non-B hepatitis is associated with a low immediate mortality, 10–50% of those infected with this virus develop a chronic hepatitis (Seeff & Hoffnagle 1977, Alter 1985) and some of these progress to cirrhosis. The cirrhosis is generally milder than that seen in alcoholics. About 10% of patients with HB develop chronic hepatitis and a proportion of these develops cirrhosis and primary hepatocellular carcinoma.

Human immunodeficiency virus

The first report of AIDS in three haemophiliacs appeared in 1982, and that of transfusion-associated AIDS was in an infant in 1983 and in adults in 1984. Most but not all recipients transfused with infected blood develop anti-HIV antibodies. Up to 1986, about 1.6% of all patients with AIDS in the USA and UK appear to have become infected from transfusion of blood or of some of its components.

Exclusion of donors carrying the virus is achieved by two methods. First, through 'self-exclusion' by appealing to all those who fall into high-risk groups to withdraw from giving blood. Secondly, by testing all donors for the presence of anti-HIV antibodies in their plasma. The average delay in the appearance of antibody after the time of infection is about 2–3 months and 95% of those infected have seroconverted by 6 months (Horsburgh *et al.* 1989). Thus donors giving blood within about 6 months of infection may not be detected. It is also possible to miss donors with only low concentrations of antibody; the incidence of individuals falling into this category is thought to be less than 1% of those infected.

Identification of HIV-positive donors is a two-stage process. Screening for antibodies is first carried out using impure antigen. In the second stage, the positive samples are retested using purified antigens by a variety of methods. Most of the samples which are positive in the initial screening are found to be false-positives, as judged by the more specific tests. In one series in the USA, 0.04% of donors were finally judged to be positive, whereas it was much lower in the UK at 0.002%. In 1986, the first full year in the UK in which the 'self-exclusion' principle and anti-HIV assays had been operative, it was calculated that only about one unit of blood in every million issued might have been infectious. Factor VIII and factor IX concentrates used in the UK today carry a negligible risk of transmitting HIV. This is not only because of the use of anti-HIV-screened plasma for their preparation but also because HIV appears to be readily inactivated by the heat-treatment such concentrates are now subjected to.

Cytomegalovirus

Cytomegalovirus is a herpes virus present in white cells and is also found free in the plasma. The incidence of infection varies in different parts of the world but in general it can be said that most people acquire the infection some time during their lives, as judged by the development of anti-CMV antibodies. As with most herpes viruses, the virus persists latently after infection and it is thought that about 1–3.5% of units of blood have the potential to transmit the virus (Tegmeier 1986). About 30% of CMV-negative patients acquire the infection after cardiac surgery; most of these are asymptomatic but about 10% develop a mononucleosis-like syndrome.

The main danger of CMV infection is in infants and immunocompromised patients. Premature neonates of low birth weight born to mothers without anti-CMV virus are especially at risk. It has been found that 25–30% of infants with these risk factors developed the infection following transfusion and about 25% of those infected died (Adler *et al.* 1983). Patients receiving transplants are also at risk and the infection is the commonest cause of death following bone marrow grafting. The only way to avoid infection in these categories of patients is to transfuse with anit-CMV-negative blood.

Other diseases

Other diseases that have been known to be transmitted by transfusion are syphilis and malaria. The prevention of transmission of syphilis is by serological testing of all donors although this will not demonstrate all those infected, since it is possible to have syphilis with negative serological tests. Another factor of importance is the storage of blood at 4°C since spirochaetes do not survive for more than a few days under these conditions. Donors with a history of malaria are not accepted.

Other hazards

Since stored blood is deficient in platelets and the labile coagulation factors (e.g. Factors V and VIII), massive blood transfusions lead to a moderate thrombocytopenia and abnormalities in the prothrombin time and activated partial thromboplastin time. When massive blood transfusions are complicated by a haemorrhagic state, bleeding may be controlled by the administration of platelet concentrates and, possibly, fresh-frozen plasma.

As each unit of blood contains about 250 mg of iron, the administration of frequent transfusions over several years results in a marked accumulation of iron in the body (transfusion haemosiderosis) and progressive wide spread tissue damage. The iron overloading can be prevented or limited by treatment with desferrioxamine subcutaneously via a pump (see p. 47).

PROCEDURE IN THE CASE OF TRANSFUSION REACTIONS

In the majority of instances it is easy to diagnose the type of transfusion reaction. Allergic reactions are obvious and, if mild, only require antihistamines. Symptoms occurring within 20 minutes of starting a transfusion are always due to red-cell incompatibility or infected blood and clearly the transfusion must be stopped. It is the occurrence of rigors and fever after 30–60 minutes which causes difficulty in the diagnosis, since some of these reactions are due to bacterial pyrogens and some are due to leucocyte, platelet or red-cell incompatibility. In these patients with delayed symptoms, the transfusion should be temporarily stopped, the blood being replaced with saline, and the patient warmed. If symptoms do not rapidly disappear, the transfusion should be abandoned and the reaction investigated further. Fortunately, reactions of this type, due to incompatibility, are only rarely fatal.

Investigation of a transfusion reaction due to incompatibility

There are two questions to answer after a suspected transfusion of incompatible blood: first, has destruction of red cells in fact taken place and, second, which antigen–antibody system was involved.

Immediately the transfusion has been stopped, a blood sample is obtained from the recipient and centrifuged; the plasma is examined for the presence of free haemoglobin and the plasma bilirubin concentration is estimated. A urine sample is also examined for the presence of haemoglobin. If incompatible cells are still present in the recipient's circulation, their presence can often be detected by serological methods. Thus, the presence of group A cells in a group O patient can be detected by the addition of anti-A which will agglutinate only A cells in the sample.

The ABO and Rh group of both the recipient and donor are checked and a cross-match repeated using the serum obtained from the recipient prior to transfusion. These tests will reveal whether the incompatibility is within the ABO system or whether it involves the D antigen of the Rh system. If the ABO and Rh(D) groups are compatible, but the cross-match shows the presence of an antibody, the specificity of the antibody can be identified by further testing against a panel of red cells of known blood-group specificity. The remains of the donor blood in the pack after every transfusion should be kept at 4°C for 48 hours so that any adverse reaction can be adequately investigated.

PLATELET AND GRANULOCYTE CONCENTRATES

Platelet concentrates are prepared either from freshly-donated units of blood or by using intermittent-flow or continuous-flow cell separators which separate platelets from blood and return the rest of the blood to the donor. They may be stored at 22°C for about 5 days. Platelet concentrates are indicated when there is clinically significant bleeding due to thrombocytopenia or a qualitative platelet defect. They should also be given prophylactically prior to surgery in a patient with a platelet count below 60×10^9/litre. Granulocyte concentrates are prepared using cell separators and may be beneficial in patients with intractable infections associated with severe neutropenia.

OBJECTIVES IN LEARNING

1 To know about the inheritance of the ABO system, and the type and distribution of associated antibody.

2 To know the distribution and mode of inheritance of the D antigen of the Rh system.

3 To know the principles involved in the selection of donor blood of suitable ABO and Rh groups for a recipient, and the principles of the cross-match, including the antiglobulin test.

4 To know the hazards of blood transfusion (incompatible blood, pyrogenic and allergic reactions, bacterial infection, citrate toxicity and transmission of disease).

5   To know how to investigate a patient suspected of receiving an incompatible transfusion.

REFERENCES

Adler S.P., Chaudrika T., Laurence L., Baggett J. (1983) Cytomegalovirus infections in neonates acquired by blood transfusion. *Paediatr Infect Dis.* **2**: 114–8

Alter H.J. (1985) Post-transfusion hepatitis: clinical features, risk and donor testing. In: *Infection Immunity and Blood Transfusion* Dodd R.Y.& Barker L. F. (Eds), pp 47–61. A.R. Liss, Inc

Choo Q., Kuo G., Weiner A.J., Overby L.R., Bradley D.W., Houghton M. (1989) Isolation of a cDNA clone derived from a blood-borne non-A, non-B viral hepatitis genome. *Science* **244**: 359–62

Horsburgh C. R., Ou C.Y., Jason J., Holmberg S.D., Longini I.M., Schable C. *et al.* (1989) Duration of human immunodeficiency virus infection before detection of antibody. *Lancet* **ii**: 637–39

Landsteiner K., Weiner A.S. (1940) An agglutinable factor in human blood recognizable by immune sera for Rhesus blood. *Proc. Soc. Exp. Biol.* (N Y) **43**: 223

Ministry of Health Memorandum (1943) Homologous serum jaundice. *Lancet* **i**: 83

Mollison P.L. (1979) Some clinical consequences of red cell incompatibility. *J.R. Coll. Physicians.* **13**: 15

Mollison P.L., Engelfriet C.P., Contreras M. (1987) *Blood Transfusion in Clinical Medicine* (8th Ed) Blackwell Scientific Publications, Oxford

Mosley J.W. (1965) The surveillance of transfusion-associated viral hepatitis. *J. Am. Med. Ass.* **193**: 1007

Pineda A.A. Taswell H.F., Brzica S.M. (1978) Delayed haemolytic transfusion reactions. An immunologic hazard of blood transfusion. *Transfusion Philad.* **18**: 1

Ramgren O., Skold E., Tanberg J. (1958) Immediate non-haemolytic reactions to blood transfusion. *Acta Med. Scand.* **162**: 211

Seeff L.B., Zimmerman H.J., Wright E.C., Finkelstein J.D., Garcia-Pont P., Greenlee H.B.(1977) A randomized, double-blind controlled trial of the efficacy of immune serum globulin for the prevention of post-transfusion hepatitis. *Gastroenterology* **72**: 111

Seeff L.B., Hoffnagle J. (1977) Leader. *Ann. Intern. Med.* **86**: 818

Stephen C.V., Martin R.C., Bourgeois-Gavardin M. (1955) Antihistaminic drugs in treatment of non-haemolytic transfusion reactions. *J. Am. Med. Ass.* **158**: 525

Tegmeier G.E. (1986) Transfusion-transmitted cytomegalovirus infections: significance and control. *Vox Sang* **51**: (Suppl 1) 22–30

Wallace J. (1977) *Blood Transfusion for Clinicians.* Churchill Livingstone, Edinburgh

RECOMMENDED READING

Race R.R., Sanger R. (1975) *Blood Groups in Man.* 6th Ed. Blackwell Scientific Publications, Oxford

Chapter 13
Basic Haematological Techniques and Normal Values

This chapter deals with the principles underlying the measurement of the most commonly determined haematological values.

HAEMOGLOBIN AND THE BLOOD COUNT

Until about two decades ago, the haemoglobin concentration per dl of blood (Hb), packed cell volume (PCV), white cell count (WBC), red cell count (RBC) and platelet count were all determined by manual methods. Today, in all diagnostic laboratories of the developed world, basic haematological parameters are measured not by manual methods but by semi-automated or fully automated electronic blood counting machines. Current fully automatedmachines provide at least the following data on every sample analysed: WBC, Hb, RBC, PCV, mean cell volume (MCV), mean cell haemoglobin (MCH), mean cell haemoglobin concentration (MCHC) and platelet count. However, two of the manual methods, namely, the cyanmethaemoglobin method for haemoglobin estimation and the Wintrobe haematocrit method (with a correction for trapped plasma) continue to be the reference methods and are used for the calibration of automated equipment.

Haemoglobin concentration

Manual method

The estimation of haemoglobin is dependent on its property of absorbing light in the yellow-green region of the visible spectrum. The blood is diluted with a solution containing potassium cyanide and potassium ferricyanide which converts all types of haemoglobin (oxyhaemoglobin, reduced haemoglobin, methaemoglobin and carboxyhaemoglobin) into the stable cyanmethaemoglobin compound. The optical density of the solution is then measured using a photo-electric colorimeter or spectrophotometer; the instrument is calibrated using a cyanmethaemoglobin standard. Haemoglobin concentration is expressed as grams of haemoglobin/dl of whole blood.

The accuracy of any particular estimate, as carried out in a routine laboratory, is difficult to assess, but is probably of the order of ±5%. The chief sources of error are failure to mix the blood adequately before sampling, and inaccurate dilution. The normal ranges for the haemoglobin concentration at different ages are given on p. 15.

Automated method

In most fully automated blood cell counters, the haemoglobin level is estimated by an adaptation of the cyanmethaemoglobin method.

Estimation of PCV

Glass tubes with an internal diameter of about 3 mm (Wintrobe haematocrit tubes) or much smaller (microhaematocrit tubes) are filled with anticoagulated blood and spun in a centrifuge under standard conditions for a fixed period. The PCV is defined as the height of the column of packed red cells expressed as a fraction of the total height of the column of packed cells plus plasma. Automated blood counting machines calculate the PCV using red cell volume data and the red cell count.

The normal range is 0.4–0.51 for men, 0.36–0.46 for women (40–51% and 36–46% using the old terminology). The PCV does not supply any more information than the haemoglobin concentration, but is useful for checking the accuracy of the latter.

Red cell count

The manual method for counting red cells involves diluting blood 1:200 in a solution containing formaldehyde and trisodium citrate (formol-citrate) and filling a Neubauer or similar type of counting chamber with the diluted blood. The chamber is placed on the stage of a microscope and at least 500 red cells are counted visually. Red cell counts determined from a total count of 500 cells are relatively inaccurate; the accuracy of the count may be increased by counting larger numbers of cells.

Modern electronic blood cell counters are capable of determining red cell counts very accurately and rapidly by counting large numbers of cells in a highly diluted sample of blood.

Estimation of red cell indices

The MCV, MCH and MCHC may be calculated from the Hb, PCV and RBC determined by manual methods according to the following equations:

$$MCV \text{ (fl)} = \frac{PCV(\text{expressed as a fraction})}{RBC \text{ (litre}^{-1})} \times 10^{15}$$

$$MCH \text{ (pg)} = \frac{Hb \text{ (g/dl)}}{RBC \text{ (litre}^{-1})} \times 10^{13}$$

$$MCHC \text{ (g/dl)} = \frac{Hb \text{ (g/dl)}}{PCV \text{ (expressed as a fraction)}}$$

Since red-cell counts obtained by manual methods are inaccurate, both the MCV and MCH determined in this way are also unreliable; the only index that can be calculated reliably is the MCHC.

Electronic cell counters vary in their method of estimating the red-cell count and red-cell size (i.e. MCV). The Coulter counters estimate these parameters on the basis of a change in electrical impedance when individual cells pass through a narrow orifice, the extent of the change being proportional to size. Other counters (Technicon, Ortho) estimate the red-cell count and MCV on the basis of the scattering of a focussed beam of light when an individual cell passes through it. Thus, electronic cell counters in current use obtain a value for MCV by measurement rather than by calculation. All of them determine the PCV from the cell volume data and the RBC. The MCH and MCHC are calculated using the equations given above.

Electronic counters have to be standardized either with blood samples in which the various haematological parameters have been determined using reference methods, or with standards provided by the manufacturers. Although such counters have greatly improved the precision of all measurements (i.e. have considerably increased reproducibility), the accuracy of the MCV, MCH and MCHC determined by such instruments (i.e. the relation between the observed result and the true value) has not yet been defined, particularly in the case of abnormal red cells.

Normal ranges in adults and common conditions in which abnormal values are found are as follows.

Mean cell volume (MCV)

The normal range is 82–99 fl (femtolitres). Values below the normal range are found in iron deficiency, thalassaemia syndromes and, sometimes, in the anaemia of chronic disorders. Values above the normal range are found in chronic alcoholism, vitamin B_{12} deficiency and folate deficiency.

Mean cell haemoglobin (MCH)

The normal range is 27–33 pg (picograms). Values below normal are found in iron deficiency, thalassaemia syndromes and in some cases of anaemia in chronic diseases.

Mean cell haemoglobin concentration (MCHC)

The normal range is 32–36 g/dl. Its main use is in the diagnosis of iron deficiency. A low MCHC is a sensitive indicator of iron deficiency only when it is calculated using a PCV determined by the haematocrit method or when it is obtained from a Technicon H1 automated cell counter. It is not a sensitive indicator of iron deficiency when obtained from a Coulter counter since under these circumstances MCHC values only fall consistently below normal when the haemoglobin is below 7 g/dl.

In apparently normal children between the ages of about 6 months and 15 years, the average values for the MCV and MCH are lower than in adults. At one time this was thought to be entirely due to a high prevalence of iron deficiency in children, but it is now clear that children with adequate iron stores have microcytic red cells and a low MCH (by adult standards) as an intrinsic feature of erythropoiesis in childhood. In children aged 1–8 years, the normal ranges for the MCV and MCH are, respectively, 70–88 fl and 24–30 pg. There is a gradual rise in the indices from the time of their lowest values at about 6 months of age; adult values are reached shortly after puberty.

White-cell count (WCC, WBC)

The manual method for determining the concentration of white cells in blood involves making a suitable dilution of whole blood, filling a counting chamber with the diluted blood and counting the white cells visually using a microscope. The diluting fluid contains acetic acid, which lyses the red cells, and a dye, such as gentian violet, to stain the white cells. This method has been superseded by electronic counting methods, which are more accurate and much quicker. In these methods, the white cells are counted, after lysing the red cells, using the same principles as for red cell counting (i.e. by measurement of electrical impedence or light scattering).

Platelet count

Several manual methods are in use. These methods involve making a suitable dilution of whole blood, filling a counting chamber and counting the unstained platelets using a phase-contrast microscope. A diluting fluid that has been found to work well is formaldehyde in sodium citrate (formol-citrate). In one method, instead of diluting whole blood, platelet-rich plasma obtained by allowing the blood to settle at room temperature is diluted; this eliminates most of the red cells from the counting chamber. Electronic methods are now available which count platelets far more quickly and with far greater accuracy than the manual methods. The normal range for the platelet count is $160-450 \times 10^9$/litre. Fully automated cell counters often count red cells and platelets in the same channel distinguishing between them on the basis of size.

RETICULOCYTE COUNT

Reticulocytes present in blood are red cells recently delivered from the marrow and contain the remains of the RNA used in haemoglobin synthesis. The reticulocyte count is the best estimate that we have of the rate of production of viable red cells (p. 27). The RNA is demonstrated by adding red cells to a solution of a dye such as brilliant cresyl blue, which precipitates the RNA as granules and filaments and also stains the precipitates. A film is then made on a slide and the proportion of reticulocytes to total red cells estimated. When the rate of red-cell production is normal, the count in adults is 1.0–3.7% in females and 0.8–2.6% in males.

It is more useful to express the reticulocyte count as the absolute concentration per litre of blood than a percentage since, when expressed as a percentage, the value is influenced by the red-cell count (or haemoglobin concentration). For instance, a value of 6% with a haemoglobin concentration of 14 g/dl would correspond to the same absolute reticulocyte count as a value of 12% with a haemoglobin concentration of 7 g/dl. In normal adults, the absolute reticulocyte count varies between 18×10^9 and 158×10^9/litre.

PREPARATION AND ROMANOWSKY STAINING OF BLOOD OR BONE MARROW SMEARS

A small drop of blood or marrow aspirate is placed on the surface of a glass slide, near one end. Another slide (spreading slide) is placed slightly in front of the drop at an angle of about 30° and is then moved back slightly so that the drop spreads at the angle between the slides. The smear is then made by rapidly moving the spreading slide forward over the surface of the first slide. The smears are air-dried and, except when required for certain cytochemical studies, are fixed in methanol. The most commonly used stains for routine morphological studies include the May-Grünwald-Giemsa stain, Wright's stain or Leishman's stain. These stains are collectively described as Romanowsky stains and contain eosin and methylene blue (plus various derivatives of methylene blue such as various Azure dyes).

THE DIFFERENTIAL LEUCOCYTE COUNT

In order to determine the relative proportion of neutrophil granulocytes, lymphocytes, etc., in the peripheral blood, their percentage distribution on a stained film is determined, assessing a minimum of 200 consecutive nucleated cells. The method is not very accurate as the distribution of various cell types on a film is not random: neutrophil granulocytes and monocytes predominate at the margins and tail of the film and lymphocytes in the centre. Fortunately, when significant deviations from normality occur in patients they are greater than the error of the differential count.

From the total white-cell count and the differential leucocyte count, the concentration of various types of white cell per unit volume of blood (absolute counts) can be calculated. In adults, the upper limit of normal is usually taken to be 11×10^9/litre of whole blood for the total white-cell count, 7.5×10^9/litre for the neutrophil granulocytes, and 3.5×10^9/litre for lymphocytes.

SERUM B$_{12}$ AND RED-CELL FOLATE ASSAYS

Serum B_{12} and red-cell folate levels can be estimated microbiologically as the organisms *Lactobacillus leichmanii* and *Lactobacillus casei* require B_{12} and folate, respectively, for growth and reproduction. The organism is incubated in the presence of serum or a haemolysate and the extent of growth estimated by the increase in turbidity, which is proportional to the amount of vitamin present. Microbiological assays are labour-intensive and prone to periodic failure. Therefore, many laboratories now measure B_{12} and folate levels using competitive protein binding radioassays. These are based on the ability of ^{57}Co-labelled B_{12} or ^{125}I-labelled pteroylglutamic acid to compete with the corresponding vitamin in serum or a haemolysate, respectively, for combination with a specific vitamin-binding protein. The normal ranges for the serum vitamin B_{12} and red-cell folate levels determined using Becton Dickinson radioassay kits are, respectively, 165–680 ng/litre and 200–800 µg/litre.

MARROW ASPIRATION AND TREPHINE BIOPSY OF THE MARROW

A sample of marrow may be obtained for examination by aspiration from the sternum (at the level of the second intercostal space) or the iliac crest. After injecting a local anaesthetic into the skin and periosteum overlying the proposed site of aspiration, a special needle (with a stylet) is gently pushed through the bone into the marrow cavity. The stylet is then removed, a syringe fitted to the needle and marrow aspirated. Drops of the aspirate are placed on glass slides and smeared. Some methanol-fixed smears are stained by a Romanowsky method and used to determine the cellularity of the marrow fragments (Plates 5–7), the myeloid/erythroid ratio (p. 29) and the percentage distribution of the various cell types present. Others must always be stained for haemosiderin using Perls' acid ferrocyanide method (Prussian blue reaction), in order to assess (a) iron stores within marrow fragments (i.e. the quantity of stainable iron present within macrophages; see Plates 9,10 and 12); and (b) the number, size and distribution of iron-containing granules within erythroblasts (Plate 11). Haemosiderin stains deep blue.

Another method of obtaining marrow for study is by trephine biopsy of the iliac crest. Here a special needle is used to obtain a core of bone and marrow. The specimen is fixed, decalcified and embedded in paraffin. Histological sections are prepared, stained with haematoxylin and eosin and studied. Some sections must also be stained by a silver impregnation method to study the distribution and quantity of reticulin fibres; this stain is important for the detection of idiopathic or secondary myelofibrosis (pp. 137 and 139).

OTHER INVESTIGATIONS

The principles underlying the prothrombin time and activated partial thromboplastin time are outlined on p. 175 and the antiglobulin test is discussed on p. 190.

SUMMARY OF NORMAL VALUES

The reference ranges (95% confidence limits) for various haematological measurements in healthy adults are shown in Table 13.1.

Table 13.1   Normal values for Caucasian adults.

Haemoglobin	
Males	13.0–17.0 g/dl
Females (non-pregnant)	12.0–15.5 g/dl
Females (pregnant)	11.0–14.0 g/dl
PCV	
Males	0.40–0.51
Females	0.36–0.46
RBC	
Males	$4.4–5.8 \times 10^{12}$/litre
Females	$4.1–5.2 \times 10^{12}$/litre
MCV	82–99 fl
MCH	27–33 pg
MCHC	32–36 g/dl
White-cell count	$4–11 \times 10^9$/litre
Platelets	$160–450 \times 10^9$ /litre
Reticulocytes	$18–158 \times 10^9$/litre
Serum iron	10–30 µmol/litre
Total iron binding capacity	50–70 µmol/litre
Serum ferritin	12–150 µg/litre
Serum B_{12}	165–680 ng/litre
Red-cell folate	200–800 µg/litre
Serum folate	3–20 µg/litre

dl = decilitre (100 ml). fl = femtolitre (1×10^{-15}litre).
pg = picogram

Index